Everything You Need to Know
About Hoarding

Are you or someone you know struggling with Hoarding Disorder, feeling ashamed or guilty about your belongings, and afraid to let them go? It's more common than you might think, affecting up to 6 per cent of the general population. But despite its prevalence, seeking help can be challenging. This new book provides a clear description of hoarding, exploring it as a symptom of other issues as well as a condition in its own right. You'll learn about different treatment options and find step-by-step guidance and tools for recovery in the self-help section. Personal narratives and case studies make this guide accessible and relatable for those affected by hoarding, as well as their loved ones and health professionals. Don't let Hoarding Disorder control your life – take the first step towards recovery today with this invaluable resource.

Dr Lynne M. Drummond is an internationally renowned psychiatrist and researcher, who has been helping people with Obsessive Compulsive Disorder (OCD) and hoarding for over 40 years. In addition to her roles as Honorary Consultant and Visiting Professor, Dr Drummond also works extensively with various charities involved with OCD and hoarding. *Everything You Need to Know About Hoarding* is her fifth book.

Laura J. Edwards is a freelance writer with an interest in making science accessible to a wider readership. She is assistant author of three books on mental health.

'Dr Drummond shines a light on the oft-neglected problem of compulsive hoarding, in this humane, clearly written, and extremely informative book. Brought to life with telling vignettes drawn from her vast clinical experience, the chapters comprehensively cover key aspects and will undoubtedly serve to enlighten all those interested in this challenging mental health problem, including healthcare professionals, the families of those with hoarding problems, and those living with hoarding themselves, instilling confidence to understand what is happening and how to seek help. Bravo!'

Naomi A. Fineberg,
Professor of Psychiatry, University of Hertfordshire and
Hertfordshire Partnership University NHS Foundation Trust

'This book will leave a powerful imprint in the reader's mind of what hoarding means and what it represents for the sufferer. For those of us who work in close proximity to people with all kinds of anxiety disorders, it is always welcoming to know that there is literature available to assist the sufferer, their loved ones, and those caring for them. All of them are so deserving of finding the right means of assistance to help in advancing a person's recovery. Helping sufferers and carers alike is a huge undertaking. To be able to do this using a self-help strategy means that the relevant support and guidance can be provided in an encouraging and structured way. This book is ideal for those who are looking for a clearer understanding of how to manage what can often be such a secret problem.'

Pamela Fox, Chairman, Triumph Over Phobia (TOP UK)

'A very informative and helpful read. Interesting history and brilliant way to bring this subject up to date. The author brings balance and perspective to hoarding. This is a read for anyone who needs to understand hoarding.'

Dave Smith, CEO, HoardingUK, www.HoardingUK.org

'Lynne Drummond is a well-known expert on obsessive compulsive and related disorders, including hoarding disorder. In this book, she provides an easy-to-read and engaging overview of hoarding, which is seen in hoarding disorders, but also in a range of other psychiatric conditions. The book will be useful to a wide audience, including those who suffer from hoarding, as well as health professionals.'

Dan Stein, Professor & Chair, Department of Psychiatry,
University of Cape Town

Everything You Need to Know About Hoarding

Lynne M. Drummond

*Honorary Consultant Psychiatrist at South West London and St George's NHS Trust
and Visiting Professor at University of Hertfordshire*

Laura J. Edwards

Freelance Writer

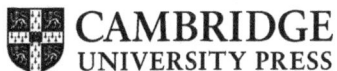

CAMBRIDGE
UNIVERSITY PRESS

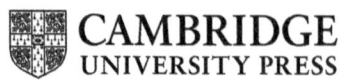

Shaftesbury Road, Cambridge CB2 8EA, United Kingdom

One Liberty Plaza, 20th Floor, New York, NY 10006, USA

477 Williamstown Road, Port Melbourne, VIC 3207, Australia

314–321, 3rd Floor, Plot 3, Splendor Forum, Jasola District Centre, New Delhi – 110025, India

103 Penang Road, #05–06/07, Visioncrest Commercial, Singapore 238467

Cambridge University Press is part of Cambridge University Press & Assessment,
a department of the University of Cambridge.

We share the University's mission to contribute to society through the pursuit of
education, learning and research at the highest international levels of excellence.

www.cambridge.org
Information on this title: www.cambridge.org/9781009466097

DOI: 10.1017/9781009466134

When citing this work, please include a reference to the
DOI 10.1017/9781009466134

First published 2025

Printed in Great Britain by CPI Group (UK) Ltd, Croydon CR0 4YY

A catalogue record for this publication is available from the British Library

A Cataloging-in-Publication data record for this book is available from the Library of Congress

ISBN 978-1-009-46609-7 Paperback

Contents

Preface

People who live with hoarding problems almost always are subject to appalling shame, embarrassment, and self-blame. For decades, hoarding has not been considered a genuine diagnosis worthy of intervention by the medical establishment, the authorities, and the general public. In the media, people who hoard have been portrayed as bad neighbours, dirty people, or people that can be laughed at and pilloried. The reaction to hoarding amongst general medical and mental health practitioners has also often been unsympathetic, with people dismissed as making "lifestyle" choices and, thus, not being offered any help. Given this situation, it is unsurprising that people with hoarding problems are fearful of asking for help and many live isolated lives resenting anyone who tries to intervene. I hope this book will serve to enlighten healthcare professionals, the families of those with relatives who have difficulty with hoarding, and most importantly those living with hoarding and Hoarding Disorder and give them confidence to understand what is happening to them and how they may seek help and start to help themselves. As I say so often, please believe there is a light at the end of the tunnel!

Brief History of the Origin of This Book

In 1979, having completed my medical degree and worked as a junior doctor in general medicine to gain higher qualifications, I started work in psychiatry on Professor Isaac Marks' Ward for people with Obsessive Compulsive Disorder (OCD). I immediately became fascinated by this condition and delighted in seeing people getting better and overcoming many of their problems. From then on, even during training, OCD and its related disorders became the main focus of my interest.

In 1985, I was appointed as a Senior Lecturer at St George's Hospital in London and a Consultant Psychiatrist in Cognitive and Behavioural Psychotherapy at what was to become South West London and St George's NHS Trust. This job included a small inpatient unit which I worked to expand and develop over the next 35 years to become the National Inpatient Service for Profound Refractory OCD and Related Disorders. At the start of my time here, conditions such as body dysmorphic disorder, hypochondriasis, health anxiety, obsessive personality, as well as hoarding, were all included under the umbrella term of "OCD". In reality, of course, we would try and develop a pragmatic way to use our skills to help these people overcome the difficulties they experienced. Medication was almost exclusively serotonin reuptake inhibiting medicines (clomipramine and SSRIs) with some additional dopamine blocking medicines used if these were not helping. Our CBT skills were more stretched as we learned to try to see what worked best. Despite writing my first book, published in 1979 with Dr Richard Stern, we did not separate out hoarding symptoms, Hoarding Disorder, and OCD.

In the early 1990s, I wrote a paper on hoarding along with some colleagues. I then discovered how difficult it was to get people to take hoarding seriously as a serious condition. Few journals were interested, with many suggesting that this was a subject for the speciality of geriatric medicine rather than psychiatry, and this was despite the relative youth of the people we described with hoarding symptoms.

In 2013, the American Psychiatric Association recognised a standalone condition of Hoarding Disorder which was included under a new classification of Obsessive Compulsive and Related Disorders. This was a huge step forward. For the first time researchers and clinicians became interested in hoarding as a real entity and as a mental health condition which, by definition, required help. At long last, we are starting to see better understanding and more research into how these problems arise and what we can do to help to relieve the suffering they cause. To this end, my books published in 2018 and 2022 on OCD contain separate sections on Hoarding Disorder.

However, what seems to so often happen now is that everyone who has hoarding problems tends to be categorised as having Hoarding Disorder. In reality, I believe that hoarding is a symptom which can be caused by a variety of physical, cognitive, developmental, and emotional factors or as an effect of other mental health conditions, as well as true Hoarding Disorder existing as a standalone condition. As I hope this book will explain, I believe there to be a huge overlap between Hoarding Disorder and other mental health conditions. Hoarding symptoms not only can arise in other conditions but the overlaps between Hoarding Disorder and some other diagnoses are also huge. Rather than listing one type of treatment to fit all, I have tried to explain how helping conditions underlying hoarding symptoms may help the individual to improve as well as offering guidance for dealing with Hoarding Disorder.

So, all this has led me to write my knowledge and to research all the current information I could find in this book, which I hope will be helpful to those living with hoarding problems, families and friends of people with hoarding issues, as well as healthcare workers, clinicians, and therapists.

Lynne M. Drummond

1

• • • • • • •

Introduction

SUMMARY

This chapter starts with a look at the concept of hoarding, beginning with what it is and how some animals and most people have a tendency to collect items beyond their immediate requirements. The distinction is made between a hoard and a collection. The types of items which are hoarded are discussed, along with a description of Animal Hoarding.

Some of the social aspects of hoarding are discussed, as it is easier for hoarding to get out of hand in a small bedsit as opposed to a large mansion with more available space. We will address the stigma of hoarding and how this can be treated by society, along with discussion of the shame and humiliation which prevents many people with hoarding problems from seeking help. This stigma can be reinforced by "helping" agencies who may view it as a "lifestyle choice" rather than a condition which requires help, and we look at the role the media has played in perpetuating the myth that hoarders should be able to deal with it themselves.

Hoarding can be regarded as a symptom rather than a distinct diagnosis and may be found in many conditions, but there is a specific condition with characteristic features known as Hoarding Disorder. Some possible causes of hoarding are then described, followed by a more detailed examination of the diagnosis of Hoarding Disorder.

Finally, the chapter examines whether hoarding only occurs in the elderly, and introduces the idea of hoarding in childhood.

What Is Hoarding?

If you look up the term "hoarding" in a dictionary, it is described as the act of keeping large amounts of food, money, or other items, and that this is often hidden from other people. Obviously, this is not a straightforward definition as most of us would prefer not to live "hand to mouth" but to store a little more for the future in case of times of greater need. Examples of this include pickling and preserving food in the abundant summer months to ensure food was available over winter in the days before freezers and refrigeration. Similarly, most of us would like to have a little more money in the bank over and above our daily outgoings if we are in a position to do so. Indeed, we are not the only animal that likes to do this. Most people will have observed squirrels burying nuts and seeds for the winter or in times of excess, only for some of these storage places to be forgotten or the contents not needed by the squirrel, and what we will see is a horse chestnut or similar sapling growing in the garden even if we are well beyond the distance where the tree would normally drop its fruit. Domestic dogs will also try and bury particularly tasty morsels of food if given a treat while not hungry at the time, and may then reappear with a maggot-infested biscuit or bone some weeks later.

Does Hoarding Matter?

We can therefore see that all of us do have a tendency to save up items and to store them for times of greater need. Such activity is usually considered prudent and a way of protecting our future. Excessive hoarding, however, can be an extremely dangerous problem even resulting in death due to the increased fire risk. If you look through a local paper, it is not unusual to see house fires reported, and if you delve a little deeper, you can find out that a high proportion of these occur in houses which are cluttered, where the occupants have obtained a large number of flammable objects. For example, it was reported that, in 2022, the London Fire Brigade attended 1036 hoarding-related fires which resulted in 186 injuries and 10 deaths.[1]

In Wales, it was reported that hoarding was responsible for 25–30 per cent of fire-related deaths.[2]

As well as fires, deaths and injuries can occur when a large quantity of items causes someone to trip and fall, or when they become trapped under an "avalanche" of possessions.

Although deaths and serious injuries are a dramatic portrayal of the difficulties that can arise from excessive hoarding, there are other more mundane effects which impact on an individual's mental and physical health.

Hoarding was not recognised as a diagnosis until 2013, but there were reports in the medical literature from the middle of the 20th century of what was described as "Diogenes Syndrome". This was mainly being described in older people and was said to consist of excessive hoarding, self-neglect, and living in squalor and unsanitary conditions. Hoarding is likely to lead to self-neglect as well as unclean conditions. If a home is full of hoarded items, then you may be unable to wash and take care of basic self-care routines. Similarly, it may be impossible to access the fridge and cooker to cook a reasonably healthy meal. Cleaning becomes impossible as objects accumulate and cover every surface. In addition, there is the possible detrimental effect of what is hoarded, so that, for example, if perishable items are contained amongst the hoard, there may be vermin including insects, maggots, rats, mice, or even other animals. Then, as a final point, if someone is spending a considerable proportion of their income on items that are hoarded or, in many cases, on renting additional space to keep their hoard, then they are likely to have a lack of money for food and heating and their health will suffer accordingly.

Jill's Story

Jill is a 50-year-old unmarried woman who lives alone in a large detached home. Despite gaining an excellent degree at university, she has never worked due to intermittent bouts of severe depression. It was during one of these episodes of depression when she was hospitalised that there were complaints from her neighbours about a smell emanating from her large suburban villa. Although Jill had never worked, she had inherited both property and money from her family and lived in an affluent part of town. Discussion was held with her and eventually, after a few weeks of discussion, she extremely reluctantly agreed that one of the therapists she trusted from the local community mental health team could accompany her on a home visit.

On entering the house, the therapist found that it was full of papers and other items with just a narrow passageway through the house. All four of the bedrooms were piled high and impossible to enter and the bath was full of objects with barely room to access the toilet. It was in the kitchen where there was the biggest surprise, as there was a strong smell and it appeared that rotting food was intermixed with the papers and other items. It was impossible for Jill to have used this space for cooking for many months or even years. As they entered the kitchen, however, a fox darted out from under the piles of accumulated items and ran though a broken window into the garden. It transpired that a family of foxes was living under the hoard in the kitchen along with rats and mice.

What Do People Typically Hoard?

While most people hoard objects which either have a practical purpose but the amount is excessive, for example, food, newspapers, etc., or which have an emotional meaning to them, for example, items from a deceased family member, others may hoard in different ways.

George's Story

George is a 45-year-old unmarried man who lives on his own in a small housing association apartment. As a young man, he had hoped to become a film critic for one of the major national newspapers, had studied journalism and film after school, and had landed a job as the arts correspondent for a small local paper. However, the local paper was bankrupt after a few years and George had been unable to find permanent work for the previous 10 years. Still having an avid interest in film, George spent money attending as many shows as possible. He also collected what he described as "film reviews" but which in fact were copies of every major newspaper which had a film section. These newspapers were piled high throughout his flat. On questioning, it appeared that George was in a considerable amount of debt, and as well as having a house full of old newspapers, he also had hired a lockup garage as well as three large containers at the local storage depot. The costs of hiring all this extra space as well as the purchase of every national newspaper every day exceeded his income, and George was pale, thin, and self-neglecting and clearly not eating sufficiently well to maintain health. He was insistent that these newspapers were a "comprehensive collection of film reviews" even though they were complete papers stacked in random piles with no attempt at classification or order, and he was unable to say where any particular review might be found.

One of the most distressing forms of hoarding is Animal Hoarding. This is most commonly seen by people working with animal charities. In these cases, the individual collects large numbers of animals who they may believe they have rescued, but in reality they have too many animals to care for appropriately and there may be many sick, neglected, or even dead animals.

Jean's Story

Jean is a 50-year-old woman who has always had a passion for animals and always had one or two dogs in her home at any one time. Ten years ago, her partner of 15 years left her for another woman, and Jean was left bereft. At approximately the same time, her elderly dog died. Friends encouraged her to adopt another dog from a dog rescue charity. At this time, Jean became fascinated by the charity and began volunteering for them. After a couple of years, she decided to set up an animal rescue in her own area. In the past, she had tried to adopt a variety of animals, but her partner had stopped her accumulating too many by insisting she place them elsewhere. Once Jean set up her own animal charity, she became more and more reclusive and was rarely seen out and about by neighbours and friends. She'd started walking her dogs very early in the morning and very late at night. Neighbours became concerned that the house was in a state of increasing dilapidation, and the noise from the animals was a cause of concern. Eventually the neighbours complained about the noise to the police. A local policeman was called, and he explained to Jean that her animals were disrupting her neighbours' sleep by the noise. Jean became very abusive on hearing this and shut the door. Being concerned about what he saw through the door, the policeman called the Royal Society for the Prevention of Cruelty to Animals (RSPCA). Two days later the police returned with the RSPCA and they tried to speak with Jean and asked to see her animals. Jean was adamant that all her animals were "fine" and that she loved them all dearly. However, the smell emanating from the house was overwhelming and a dog that was seen in the doorway appeared emaciated. The RSPCA officer informed Jean that he was concerned about her animals and would like to see all of them. At first Jean denied anyone entry but, when it became clear to her that the police and RSPCA were looking to collect evidence for a court case, she reluctantly let them in. They found she had 30 dogs in a tiny space, and the floors and carpets were covered in faeces. All the dogs looked unhealthily thin. When asked when the dogs had been seen by a veterinarian, Jean said that she had not taken them. She tearfully expressed how much she loved her dogs and begged the RSPCA not to take them from her as she believed she had a special bond with each and every dog and that no one else could care for them in the way she did. Eventually it was agreed that the RSPCA could return with a veterinarian. Over the next few weeks, plans were made to encourage Jean to agree to let some of her dogs be rehomed elsewhere. Sadly this occurred by threatening her with court action, which would have meant prosecution and her losing the right to keep any animals.

Sadly, unlike with object hoarding, most people who hoard animals are still dealt with via the courts as many are unwilling to work with the animal charities, so the only course of action to protect the animals is via legal pathways. Similarly, very few people with animal hoarding issues are seen by mental health services; therefore, there is little research in this area. Most descriptions and research regarding Animal Hoarding have been published in veterinarian publications, and is animal-focussed.

Is There Any Difference between a Collection and a Hoard?

Some people collect items which may be of little interest and perceived as being of low value to others. For example, a collection of railway timetables, stamps, football stickers, etc., will be seen as very valuable to those who are interested in the area but not to other people. The question then arises as to what makes a collection different from a hoard.

In a collection, even if it is large and unwieldy, there is usually some kind of categorisation so that the collector can find an individual item without too much difficulty. On the other hand, a hoard is generally chaotic without any real categorisation or ability of the individual to easily find a particular item.

For example, in the story of George in this chapter, we described a man who collected huge quantities of newspapers due to his interest in film reviews. However, these were huge piles of newspapers and were not categorised in any particular way. Contrast this with James, who is also interested in film reviews. James also collects all the major newspapers on a daily basis. He reads the film reviews and cuts out the relevant articles. These articles are then put into plastic pouches and filed by date. In both cases, the items collected are film reviews from newspapers, and in both cases, these would be considered worthless and maybe excessive by others who do not share this interest. The main difference lies in the categorisation and ability to find specific articles. Even if George had cut out the various reviews from the newspapers, unless he had organised them they would still create a chaotic mess, even if it would have taken him longer to fill up so much space.

So we can see that organisation to enable retrieval is a characteristic of a collection rather than a hoard.

Socioeconomic Aspects of Hoarding

Obviously, there are differences in the ability of someone to run out of space if they live in smaller spaces than if they live in a large mansion. Similarly, it is easier for someone on a lower income to get into debt in trying to maintain their hoard by either excessive purchasing of items or by needing to rent additional space to store them. In the case of Animal Hoarding, a very rich person may be able to accumulate a large number of animals but still afford to maintain them in a good state of health.

Differences also arise about concern about hoarding. It is much more likely that an individual who lives in close proximity to others, such as in a block of flats, will be reported to the authorities for hoarding issues than those who live more isolated lives in larger detached properties.

All of this means that we may have a skewed idea of hoarding, as those with lower incomes may be more likely to be reported to the authorities and be seen by mental health services.

Due to the shame associated with hoarding, few people come forward for help. Most people with hoarding difficulties are discovered by neighbours, friends, and family or after an event such as a fire or complaints about smell or objects blocking outside spaces.

Stigma Associated with Hoarding

Unfortunately, huge stigma exists about hoarding. While this is sadly true of many mental health conditions, it seems to be particularly true about hoarding. As a condition, Hoarding Disorder was not officially recognised as a mental illness until 2013. There is still a tendency to blame people who hoard and to portray them as lazy, slovenly, and dirty. This is hugely unfair and leads to huge suffering on the part of the person with hoarding difficulties.

In the media, there have been many television programmes which portray hoarding as a joke, or someone who hoards as being deliberately difficult. Add to this that, until recently, many mental health services would consider hoarding as a lifestyle choice rather than a disorder.

Given this stigma, it is unsurprising that many people with hoarding problems are unwilling to seek help and unable to admit to a problem.

What Are the Causes of Hoarding?

Although since 2013 there has been a diagnosis of Hoarding Disorder, it is important to remember that hoarding is a symptom which can be present in a range of physical, emotional, and mental disorders.

Hoarding may arise due to physical problems with discarding items, for example, lack of mobility meaning inability to discard items; lack of ability and motivation to face the problem, for example, severe depression, substance addiction; an inability to sort and categorise items, for example, issues such as dementia or certain types of learning disability; fear of harming oneself or others by discarding items, for example, Obsessive Compulsive Disorder (OCD) as well as being a prominent feature of Obsessive Compulsive Personality Disorder (OCPD) and, of course, Hoarding Disorder itself.

There is further discussion of conditions which may result in hoarding but not be due to a true Hoarding Disorder in the next two chapters.

What Is Hoarding Disorder?

In all healthcare disciplines, it is important that people understand what is meant by a particular diagnosis so that they can communicate with each other, research specific topics, and be fairly certain that the same condition is being researched. There are two main producers of these lists of diagnoses, which feature lists of symptoms of what is required to make a diagnosis of any particular condition. The World Health Organization produces a list known as the *International Classification of Diseases*, with the most recent version (the 11th Revision, ICD-11) being released in 2022. Another list is the American Psychiatric Association's *Diagnostic and Statistical Manual of Mental Disorders*, 5th Edition (DSM-5), which was published in 2013 and has had several updates and revisions since then.

In 2013, the concept of Hoarding Disorder was included in the newly published DSM-5, which was launched in May of that year. To produce the list, groups of experts in different fields of study come together to agree on lists of symptoms and diagnoses. DSM-5 introduced the new category of Hoarding Disorder, which is included in a section headed Obsessive Compulsive and Related Disorders.

This addition of Hoarding Disorders as a separate diagnosis is important, as until then, anyone with the symptom of hoarding was automatically placed in the diagnosis of OCD or Obsessive Compulsive Personality Disorder (OCPD), and there was no real research examining the characteristics, treatment, and response to treatment of people with Hoarding Disorder. Over a decade later, we now have much more information about this condition.

Hoarding Disorder is described in DSM-5 as persistent difficulty in throwing or giving away items irrespective of their real value to others. This difficulty in parting with objects is due to an urge to save items, and distress caused by parting with them. This difficulty in discarding leads to a cluttered environment which means that it is impossible or very difficult to use the rooms in a house for their intended use, for example, the bath is full of items or there is no space to sit in the living area. The hoarding causes difficulty in carrying out normal activities, or places the individual or others in danger. The hoarding should not be explained by another medical or psychological condition, for example, brain injury or OCD.

Beatrice's Story

Beatrice is a 75-year-old unmarried woman who lives in a housing association property. The housing association became involved when neighbours complained that boxes in the communal area outside her flat were creating a nuisance and limiting their ability to move around or to reach the fire escape in the event of an emergency evacuation. The fire service was asked to pay a visit and to assess the situation. When they arrived at a prearranged time together with representatives from the housing association, Beatrice was initially helpful and agreed that she would move the boxes. However, when it was suggested that she let the group into her flat, she became angry and refused. She was told that it was in her rental agreement that the landlords could ask to enter the property if necessary at a prearranged time. A date was therefore set for a week away.

At this follow-up appointment, Beatrice was defensive and still refused admission. After very lengthy discussions, she did however agree that she would attend an appointment at her general practitioner (GP) and ask for a mental health assessment.

Her GP knew Beatrice well and was aware that she had been evicted by several private landlords in the past. She had always lived alone and was extremely reluctant to let anyone into her property, which was piled high with papers, books, and magazines. On previous attempts to help her clear her living space, she had claimed that losing her possessions was equivalent to being raped by the mental health team. She had no significant mental health history, although her GP had been concerned about her low mood in the past when she had been evicted. For many years, she had worked as a clerk but retired at the age of 60 years, and it appeared that her hoarding issues became worse after retirement as she would spend long periods of time perusing second-hand book shops and purchasing magazines, old papers, and books. The GP described how she had a good relationship with Beatrice but that, in general, Beatrice was a loner who avoided the company of others.

Is Hoarding Purely an Issue of Older Adults? What about Hoarding in Children?

We have already discussed how there has been a lack of research in hoarding in adults over the years and how often it was included under OCD even when there was no evidence of clear obsessions and compulsions.

When adults with significant hoarding problems and Hoarding Disorder are questioned, they frequently say that they first started to hoard items in childhood. There are no good studies of Hoarding Disorder as a standalone issue in children.

Childhood hoarding is unlikely to be a major problem, as parents will tend to oversee discarding and clearing of their living areas. Also, for any items that need to be purchased, parents or guardians are likely to be in control of the money that a child receives. This means it is unlikely that children will present for help with a serious hoarding problem. In a study from Turkey, the authors asked parents of schoolchildren to complete a screening questionnaire for hoarding problems. This was followed up by interviews. It was discovered that almost 1 per cent of the children demonstrated significant hoarding behaviours. Of those who had hoarding behaviours, girls appeared to be three times more likely than boys to be diagnosed with hoarding, and over half had evidence of another mental disorder.[3]

Children who hoard have been noted to be more likely to have diagnoses of Attention Deficit Hyperactivity Disorder (ADHD), OCD, or anxiety disorders.

Even though there is little research about children with hoarding problems, it is clear that it is an important issue which should not be overlooked. We know that, in general, if childhood mental illness is addressed early, the child has a generally good prognosis and is less likely to have severe problems in adult life. Greater awareness of the possibility of hoarding difficulties in childhood and adolescence and encouraging concerned parents to seek help is an important first step. Most adolescents can be untidy and may be lazy in throwing items away, leading to a disorganised and cluttered bedroom. There is a difference, however, in that most teenagers would be quite happy to discard items which they don't need. Of course, some items that may be collected, such as football stickers, seem to have little actual value to someone who does not follow football, but will be considered very precious by the individual collector. Parents need to decide whether they have a child with a normal disorganisation and passion for a particular study, or a more generalised issue with discarding of items. The following case story highlights the difference.

Wayne's Story

Wayne is a 14-year-old adolescent who loves football. Most of his conversation involves talking about football and he enjoys playing for his school team. Wayne's mother has two younger boys and separated from their father 7 years ago. Their father visits the children at weekends and takes them out, but he does not have space for the children to stay overnight. Their mother works as a school dinner lady but has more recently also started another job as a cleaner to try and improve their finances. In order to do this, she has asked the children to help with light housework in their own rooms. The younger boys share a bedroom, but Wayne has a room of his own. His mother became increasingly annoyed by the state of Wayne's bedroom. He never brought down dirty clothes for washing and his football kit was left for days and worn multiple times until his mother insisted he could not go to football with his smelly kit. In addition, there were half-eaten packets of crisps and biscuits, as well as dirty cutlery and crockery, strewn all over his bedroom.

His mother told Wayne he was not allowed to go to football training or matches until he cleared his bedroom. She warned him that she would inform his school football coach of the reason for his non-attendance. Although Wayne complained and shouted initially, the threat of his mother going to speak with the football coach meant that Wayne tidied his bedroom. It is far from perfectly neat and tidy, but if it starts to get out of hand again, his mother just has to remind him that she is happy to visit the football coach!

SUMMARY

- Some animals and all people often collect more items than is necessary for their immediate use, for example, pickling of vegetables to use over winter.

- Hoarding is an important cause of both ill health and even death by accidents and fires.

- Some people hoard a wide variety of objects and papers and some may hoard animals.

- Poorer people are more likely to be diagnosed with hoarding difficulties, whereas better-off people may be more able to hide the extent of their hoarding problems by purchasing/renting more space, and also because they may not live as close to others.

- Portrayal of hoarding in the media has frequently not been helpful and has undoubtedly added to the stigma associated with hoarding and the resultant shame, humiliation, and embarrassment experienced by those with a hoarding problem.

- Various physical, mental, neurodevelopmental, and psychological issues can result in hoarding as a symptom.

- Hoarding Disorder as a condition not caused by any other physical or mental condition was first fully described in 2013; therefore, there is little reliable research into the condition prior to this time.

- Hoarding Disorder involves accumulation of large amounts of items which the person has difficulty in throwing or giving away. This excessive accumulation results in difficulty using the living space fully due to accumulated clutter.

- Although often described in older adults, hoarding probably has its roots in childhood in most people. Living with others tends to reduce the side effects of hoarding, and it is later in life when more people are living alone that hoarding is seen.

2

• • • • • • •

When Does Hoarding Arise?

In this chapter, we will discuss that as well as being the main feature necessary for the diagnosis of Hoarding Disorder, hoarding can also occur as a symptom in many other physical and mental conditions. We will discuss clinical stories of people who have had difficulties with hoarding but will demonstrate how a different type of approach is needed to help them overcome their problems from that described for pure Hoarding Disorder. There will then be a brief examination of the overlap between trauma and neurodiversity and hoarding, as well as a brief description of the concept of Diogenes Syndrome in the elderly.

What Can Cause or Result in Hoarding?

As we mentioned in Chapter 1, although there is a specific condition known as Hoarding Disorder, hoarding can occur in a whole range of conditions and situations. Hoarding can be a symptom of a range of physical, emotional, and/or psychological states and does not on its own constitute a diagnosis of Hoarding Disorder.

Table 2.1 lists some of the potential causes of the symptom of hoarding. Please note that these are not exclusive; there may be many other reasons for hoarding to develop, and often a combination of factors can lead to problematic hoarding.

Table 2.1 Possible Causes of Hoarding
(please note these are examples and not meant to be exhaustive)

Primary cause	Examples of the issues	Examples of the possible causes	Notes and likely major cause of hoarding
Physical impairments	Inability to clear and discard items due to physical disability	Arthritis, movement disorders, paralysis, making the actual act of disposal problematic. Also heart or lung condition making the act of disposal difficult	Difficulty in the act of disposal of items in most cases. Pain may reduce ability to sort and dispose of items
	Extreme tiredness and fatigue leading to difficulty in sorting of items	Conditions such as chronic fatigue syndrome and long COVID leading to mental confusion and low levels of energy; chronic heart or lung disease	As above but also some "brain fog" in some conditions making organisation difficult
Brain damage	Damage to areas responsible for making decisions and choices	Brain damage following a road traffic accident or a major incident with severe head trauma. Some types of learning disability can make the organisation and categorisation of items difficult and result in hoarding of objects Can be seen following a stroke or cerebrovascular accident in these areas of the brain	May be difficulty in making decisions, difficulty in organisational skills, or brain fog

Primary cause	Examples of the issues	Examples of the possible causes	Notes and likely major cause of hoarding
	Progressive damage to brain tissue	Dementia	Organisation difficulty plus difficulty in decision making. Early dementia is likely to be a cause in what was previously described as Diogenes Syndrome with the triad of hoarding, self-neglect, and living in squalor despite no obvious cognitive impairments
Psychological disorders	Affective disorders	Depression	Brain fog and lack of motivation and drive
		Hypomania/ Bipolar Disorder	When feeling extremely exuberant and energised, activities such as cleaning and clearing are not attended to
	Drug and/or alcohol misuse disorders	Alcohol or other psychotropic drug dependency and misuse	Lack of motivation and drive for anything outside of the drug-seeking behaviour
	Obsessive Compulsive and Related Disorders	OCD	In OCD, there may be difficulty disposing of items due to obsessive thoughts and fears, e.g., reluctance to throw items away due to fear of contaminating others

Table 2.1 (Cont.)

Primary cause	Examples of the issues	Examples of the possible causes	Notes and likely major cause of hoarding
			Pure Hoarding Disorder is also common in OCD and other OC-related disorders as an independent secondary diagnosis
		Hoarding Disorder	New diagnosis since 2013, associated with strong attachment to the hoarding of objects not seen in the above causes
	Personality Disorder	Obsessive Compulsive Personality Disorder (OCPD)	Hoarding is listed as one of the characteristics of OCPD, along with living a frugal life, miserliness, perfectionism. There is a huge overlap with Hoarding Disorder, which may be a reflection of the same issue. However, not all people with OCPD hoard
	Other "neurodevelopmental" disorders	Autistic Spectrum Disorder	Hoarding and also other traits associated with OCD are common in people with autism
	Eating disorders	Anorexia Nervosa	Despite the fact that many people who

Primary cause	Examples of the issues	Examples of the possible causes	Notes and likely major cause of hoarding
			work with people with eating disorders report that hoarding is often found in those with anorexia, there are few descriptions of this in the literature. People with anorexia may hide food to avoid eating it, which may appear as hoarding, but in addition a sizeable number of people with anorexia additionally have features of OCPD or autism, and hoarding may be a feature of both of these
	Psychological trauma	Emotionally Unstable Personality Disorder (EUPD), Post-Traumatic Stress Disorder (PTSD)	Hoarding is commonly experienced in those who had a traumatic and deprived early upbringing. This may result in hoarding as a major feature. The research on the exact relationship between traumatic life events and hoarding is somewhat contradictory and difficult to fully interpret, although it is likely that trauma is associated with hoarding behaviours

How Does the Symptom of Hoarding Develop?

In order for a hoard to develop, there must be an issue with one of the following:

- **Acquisition** (buying, obtaining, or collecting items)
- **Classification** (sorting and storing items)
- **Disposal** (getting rid of those items which are either no longer necessary or more than the person needs)

We will now discuss these one by one, with examples to explain why someone may find themselves in a situation where they have a huge number of objects.

Acquisition

Some people collect and obtain more items than can be reasonably stored in their living environment. The socioeconomic aspects of this have already been discussed in Chapter 1, so that someone who lives in a large mansion is going to take longer before their hoarding becomes a problem than someone living in a studio flat. People may obtain a large number of items for a variety of reasons. For example, some individuals find that shopping lifts their mood, and they therefore have great joy and excitement from excessive shopping and acquiring a large number of items. Whereas someone with Hoarding Disorder would then have difficulty disposing of items, someone who just enjoyed shopping may not have the same sentimental attachment, and may find it relatively easy to clear a space once they have the motivation and energy to do so. Because such shopping sprees are often associated with depression and low mood, the whole task of sorting and disposing of unwanted items becomes difficult or impossible. The real-life story of Jackie illustrates this type of difficulty.

Jackie's Story

Jackie is a 40-year-old nursing assistant working in a busy Accident and Emergency Department. Although she really loves her job, she has found that the pressure of work, particularly during and after the pandemic, has taken its toll, and she regularly returns from work exhausted and with little energy to do much else. Whereas she's previously had an active social life mixing with married and unmarried friends, over the past few years Jackie has become increasingly isolated and began making excuses to avoid invitations. Inevitably, the number of invitations then started to reduce. Living alone and not having a current partner, Jackie found herself feeling increasingly low in mood and with no one to talk to. At work, the demands of her job were such that she had little time to talk to colleagues, and if she did, she found that many of them were similarly stressed and feeling undervalued. Jackie had little money but still found that her greatest pleasure was going and buying new clothes from the local discount store and charity shops. She would return home feeling happier and try the clothes on, only to leave them in an increasing pile in her bedroom. The temporary lift in mood from buying the clothes was soon replaced by a guilty feeling that she could not afford these and that they were a waste of money. Over time, as she found she was less hungry than usual, Jackie began to eat less and buy more clothes as she lost weight. One day, her sister, Jenny, unexpectedly visited her at home, so Jackie was not prepared for the visit. Recently, she had made excuses as to why she should meet her sister outside of her home. Jenny was shocked by how unwell and desperately thin Jackie was looking, and was then horrified by the state of the flat, where there were piles of clothing, meaning that it was difficult to sit on a chair or lie on the bed without moving items. At first Jackie was defensive and refused to accept anything was wrong with her, but eventually she agreed with Jenny that they would both go and see her general practitioner (GP).

The GP insisted that she take at least 4 weeks off work and prescribed an antidepressant to Jackie as well as arranging for her to see the practice counsellor. Eventually, it took 3 months for Jackie to fully improve, recover, and regain some weight. She easily then sorted out the clothes and just kept the ones she needed and liked. She returned to work after this time and, although very busy, made sure she made time to visit and socialise with friends.

Sometimes excessive acquisition can happen very quickly, such as when a family member dies and an individual suddenly inherits a large number of items. In this case, there is often some emotional attachment to the memories associated with the items, which can make it difficult to deal with.

Billy's Story

Billy is a 35-year-old accountant who lives on his own in a two-bedroomed flat in the city centre. Five years, ago his parents were killed in a road traffic accident. This event was clearly very traumatic to Billy and also his younger sister. After a court case in which the driver of the other vehicle was convicted of dangerous driving, Billy and his sister, Daisy, obtained probate for their parents' estate and began sorting out their belongings. Daisy was far more "ruthless" about what they should keep of her parents' belongings, and consequently Billy had many more boxes of items which he intended to sort through in his flat. However, 4 years on from obtaining probate, Billy still had boxes unopened and making it difficult to move freely around his small flat. He was frightened to open the boxes as he knew this would be painful and bring back memories, but he also realised that he was avoiding this issue.

Eventually, at Daisy's request, their aunt agreed to visit Billy and help him sort through the belongings. Billy was close to his aunt but was reluctant at first to do this, fearing what emotions might result from seeing items he so strongly associated with his parents. However, Billy agreed to arrange a week of leave from work and for his aunt to come and stay. The first evening that she arrived, Billy and his aunt sat and talked about many happy family holidays they had all spent together since he had been a small child. This was one of the first times that Billy had cried since his parents' funerals. Being the last remaining man of the family, Billy had tried to keep strong by not showing his emotions and burying himself into work. His aunt talked to him about how they would go through the boxes and decide what would be best for each item, which would also include thinking about what his parents would have wished.

Billy was very apprehensive but agreed to start the next day by opening the first box. This was a very slow process as many items made the pair recall stories and they found themselves crying but also laughing at the memories as they made the decisions about what to do with each item. Some items were kept but many had little use to Billy and were passed on to go to the charity shop and yet others were in too much of a state of disrepair and needed to be discarded or recycled. The thought of some of the items such as clothes and kitchen utensils helping someone else was a comfort to Billy, and he found he enjoyed the process of reminiscing and sorting, even if some of the memories were painful to him.

The stories of Billy and Jackie both demonstrate symptoms of hoarding due to excessive acquisition without appropriate discarding of items. Neither of these examples demonstrates the features of a Hoarding Disorder, as both were able to sort and discard items once offered help. In Billy's case, he did feel attachment to many of the items due to his association of these items with his parents, but he felt able to let go of many of these and to just keep a few important items to remember them by. Someone with Hoarding Disorder would have usually had far more difficulty in letting go of the items following such a sad and traumatic event.

Classification

As well as being able to control acquisition of items to prevent or control hoarding, an individual needs to be able to classify items in their mind. In other words, they need to be able to decide whether or not the item is worth keeping and if so to what purpose.

This kind of classification is dependent on what we describe as the "executive" areas of the brain. The main areas involved are the frontal and temporal regions, that is, the parts of the brain near the forehead and at the front sides of the head. In certain neurological conditions such as a stroke, often called a "cerebrovascular accident" by medical staff, this function can become impaired. Another common cause of interference with these areas in the brain is dementia, and the most frequent is Alzheimer's or Senile Dementia. In such cases, the loss of or failure to develop the ability to sort and classify items can be seen.

Effie's Story

Euphemia, who is known as "Effie", is a 98-year-old lady who until recently was living alone in a three-bedroomed house in the suburbs. Effie had been a nurse and had worked in child health all her life until retirement. Ten years ago, she lost her husband of 53 years when he died following a fall. Always fiercely independent, Effie refused offers from her grown-up children to go and live with them and insisted she could manage on her own. Reluctantly, she agreed to have a cleaner but otherwise she insisted on no additional help. Over the past year, her cleaner reported to Effie's family, who all lived overseas, that she was concerned that Effie was becoming increasingly forgetful. Her daughter Suzie decided that it was time to go and stay with Effie and to assess what was the truth about her mother. Effie had always been a loving parent and would have welcomed the chance of having her daughter to stay, and in the past she would have spent several days cooking and freezing Suzie's favourite meals so that they could maximise their time together without having to cook too frequently. Therefore, Suzie was surprised and concerned when Effie seemed less than enthusiastic when she discussed her plans to come and stay in the family home.

When Suzie arrived at the home she was immediately struck by how untidy the place was compared with usual, but dismissed this as being due to her mother getting older and having less energy to clean up. However, when she went with her mother to make a cup of tea, she became more concerned. Effie seemed to be struggling with making the tea. She boiled the kettle but forgot where the teapot was and then filled it with water without adding any tea. Not wishing to think otherwise, Suzie decided it was just that Effie was excited and tired by her visit.

Over the next few days, however, Suzie became increasingly concerned. She discovered cupboards rammed full of a variety of things, and packets of out-of-date biscuits stashed under Effie's bed and in the wardrobe. The bathroom was packed with various items of clothing which the cleaner had placed in cardboard boxes but had never been sorted. From being a very efficient, clean, and tidy person, Effie now lived in chaos. She had clearly been buying her favourite biscuits and hiding them throughout the house, and some of these packets were

2 years after their sell-by date. In addition, it became apparent that Effie was also buying a large amount of clothes and then leaving her dirty washing. Although her cleaner found some of these items, many were left pushed away in unusual places such as the back of the airing cupboard. When Suzie went into the garage to find some secateurs to prune the roses, she was greeted by a mass of objects strewn up to the ceiling. It appeared that prior to a visit from her cleaner, Effie would just throw any items she found into the garage. Consequently, it was full of clean and dirty clothes, half eaten biscuits, and had attracted mice and rats who were feasting on the food. In addition, Suzie had noticed that, whereas her mother was happy to talk about family holidays that had happened years ago, she had difficulty in remembering events that happened recently.

Suzie arranged for a joint appointment with her GP and also arranged for a skip, some de-clutterers, and a visit from pest controllers to sort out the garage. At the GP appointment, Effie was asked what she had eaten for breakfast. She replied "poached eggs on toast and a cup of tea". Suzie pointed out that in reality she had refused all breakfast and had later been found by Suzie eating a packet of stale biscuits. When asked what she had done over the past week, Effie gave a description of visiting friends, attending church, and going for walks, even though her daughter had been with her and they had not done any of the activities stated and her mother had been reluctant to leave the house. It became clear that Effie, who was always a very bright and clever woman, was suffering from quite severe memory loss but was managing to hide this from many people by answering with socially appropriate but fabricated answers. It also became clear that Effie was living mainly on biscuits and had bought little else for several months. The GP arranged for a home visit from the local older adults mental health assessment unit. After various tests, it was shown that Effie was suffering from an Alzheimer's type of dementia. After a family meeting, it was agreed that it would be better for Effie to move into a home where she would be cared for. Effie was adamant that she didn't wish to do this. Suzie also took her to visit several care homes, and Effie eventually saw one which she felt was a hotel and agreed to move in there.

Effie remains very happy in the "hotel" and has made friends with other residents and is popular with staff.

Disposal

If an individual is not able to dispose of items which are no longer useful then hoarding can occur. Problems with disposal may arise in various physical conditions where a person may not be able to go to the rubbish bin easily. This problem can also arise due to psychological conditions such as OCD where, for example, fear that rubbish is "contaminated" and could cause harm to others may lead to difficulty in throwing items away. Similarly, in a person with OCD, fear of losing something important may mean that the person checks excessively before throwing anything away. The time taken to do these checks and rechecks results in a hoard accumulating as the task becomes overwhelming. Other people may appear to hoard because they are so low in mood that any attempt to sort and dispose of items appears overwhelming. Also, someone who is experiencing hypomania may spend money and acquire a large number of items that they cannot afford, but then disposing of rubbish and unneeded items seems too trivial and is not attended to.

Sameer's Story

Sameer is a 32-year-old actor who has had a successful career with small parts in television series and TV adverts, as well as theatre. He was diagnosed with Bipolar Disorder at the age of 22 years, but in general, this is well controlled on medication.

Last year, he had been particularly busy and was working on several projects simultaneously. This workload meant that he often was sleeping for only a few hours a night and was unable to maintain the routine which he'd previously found useful. Initially no one noticed any change in Sameer but he began to feel happy, exuberant, and successful. This more outgoing side of his personality attracted more people to spend time with him. In addition, Sameer started to be the one who would pick up the bill when the cast went out for drinks and meals. His clothes became more flamboyant, colourful, and also expensive with him buying many designer items of clothing. His popularity seemed to grow, and he attracted many people who started to follow him around and partake of his largesse; this concerned his old friends who had known him for years, but Sameer did not want to listen to their warnings. Over a short time though, he began to not seem as happy but to become increasingly irritable if anyone thwarted him. This culminated in one day when, surrounded by acquaintances in a nightclub in London, he decided to buy everyone champagne. One man on a neighbouring table refused this and an argument broke out which ended in Sameer hitting the man. The police were called and arrested him. It became very quickly obvious to the police that Sameer was not in a normal mental state as he was chatty and laughing whilst they were arresting him. They thought he might have ingested a stimulant such as cocaine but decided to take him on a police section to the local mental health assessment unit. It was soon discovered that Sameer was known to mental health services and he was admitted to hospital. After treatment for a few weeks, a Community Mental Health Nurse went back to Sameer's flat with him. The apartment was in a dreadful state with expensive clothes strewn everywhere amidst unopened mail and unwashed plates and food. The nature and extent of Sameer's debts were discovered and he was given advice about how to sort these via the local Citizens Advice Bureau.

Sameer now has a list of symptoms to watch out for which may mean he is at risk of becoming hypomanic and has given these to his close friends who he agrees should contact his Community Psychiatric Nurse if they become concerned.

In the story of Sameer, he had a history of suddenly acquiring a large number of items but also had issues with classifying and sorting his possessions and then did not dispose of items appropriately because he was preoccupied with other things.

This mixture of issues is found in many people with hoarding symptoms.

Diogenes Syndrome

Diogenes was a philosopher who lived in the 4th century BC who rejected the idea of possessions and promoted ideas of self-sufficiency. He slept rough, and it is sometimes claimed he slept in an empty barrel and existed on food handouts. The main tenets of his teaching were for a lack of shame, to be outspoken, and contempt of society and social organisations.

The idea of Diogenes Syndrome first appeared in the geriatric medicine literature in the 1970s and was described as elderly people living in a state of extreme self-neglect and squalid unhygienic surroundings, self-isolation from society, refusal to seek help or acknowledge a problem, and the accumulation of a large number of unusual or unnecessary items. It is not recognised as a formal diagnosis but is still used occasionally as a term in medicine and psychiatry of older adults.

In a study of people in East Baltimore, USA, 15 per cent of elderly people with moderate and severe social breakdown were found to have dementia. This rate of dementia is twice what would be expected for adults of a similar age.[1] Another study of people with frontotemporal dementia (as described in the story of Euphemia/Effie earlier in this chapter) found that 36 per cent had the symptoms of Diogenes Syndrome.[2]

Overall there seems to be little merit in maintaining the label of Diogenes Syndrome, as it does not seem to be related to any specific pathology. By definition, it appears to be applied only to the elderly and may be found in those with Hoarding Disorder, dementia, OCD, and a range of other conditions.

Association between Psychological Trauma and Hoarding

We have already noted that there is limited research examining the possible causes of hoarding. The strong emotional attachment most people with Hoarding Disorder feel towards inanimate objects has led to speculation about early experiences and bonding to adults. Studies have shown that there are three main ways in which traumatic events may worsen or even potentially cause a hoarding problem.

The intense attachment people with Hoarding Disorder have been described to have to the items in their hoard which would often be perceived by others as rubbish or of little value has been one of the hallmarks of this condition. There has been intense speculation that this excessive attachment to objects may result from an unhappy and deprived upbringing, a lack of emotion and love in the family, or traumatic life events, with a central theme of loss and deprivation. There is limited research in this area, but overall it appears that people with Hoarding Disorder report a greater number of traumatic events in their lives and a greater range of types of traumatic events. The relationship between Hoarding Disorder and Trauma will be examined in Chapter 3.

Neurodiversity and Hoarding

It has been increasingly recognised that, along with differences in physical appearance, individuals vary in the way in which their brains process information. These conditions are, of course, on a spectrum and so can vary from mild forms through to severe. Examples of common types of neurodiversity include:

- Attention Deficit Hyperactivity Disorder (ADHD)

People with ADHD usually have shorter attention spans, can be restless and fidgety, and may be impulsive.

- Dyslexia

This is sometimes known as word blindness. It usually relates to difficulty in relating words and sounds with the letters and words on a page or a computer screen.

- Dyspraxia

This refers to a difficulty in coordinating movements. Often movements can appear awkward or clumsy, and more effort may be required to perform movements others would find easy. There is usually poor spatial awareness, so trips, falls, and bruises are common.

- Dyscalculia

This refers to difficulty in performing tasks related to numbers and counting.

- Autistic Spectrum Disorder (ASD)

People with ASD vary widely in their presentation and, of course, being on a spectrum means that there is a wide variety of ways in which this may impact on the person's life. In general, people with ASD have difficulties with social communication, often finding it difficult to interpret the emotions of others from their expressions, actions, or words. For this reason, they are often socially isolated to some extent and may find it more difficult to make friends. They may also have extreme interests and thus may be prone to collect items. High sensitivity to certain or loud sounds, strong flavours and scents, or specific textures can mean that they avoid the external world more and prefer to keep to environments they know and can predict. People with ASD may also have features of any of the other neurodiversities listed above. The ability of some people with autism to concentrate intensely on specific things of interest has meant that sometimes ASD has been viewed by the person as an advantage rather than a disadvantage.

The way in which neurodiversity can impact and co-exist with problematic hoarding will be discussed in Chapter 6.

KEY POINTS

- Hoarding is a symptom or cluster of symptoms which can be found in a wide range of physical, psychological, and developmental conditions.
- There is a separate syndrome of Hoarding Disorder which has some different features when compared with hoarding secondary to another problem.

- Problematic hoarding may arise from:
  - Excessive acquisition of items (e.g., buying more than necessary, collecting items such as leaflets).
  - Problems with classification and sorting (if people cannot classify and arrange items they may develop into a messy hoard where nothing can be found).
  - Problems in discarding objects (this may be due to extreme attachment to an item, or purely inability to get to an area where the items can be discarded).
- In the past, elderly people who were found to socially isolate themselves, live in squalid surroundings, neglect their own health and hygiene, and hoard large numbers of items, or who had several of these symptoms, were described as having Diogenes Syndrome. This is not an official diagnosis and does not seem to have any particular merit in describing individuals, as this combination may be found in people suffering from a range of difficulties.
- Psychological trauma can be seen frequently in people with problematic hoarding. This can be long-standing deprivation, neglect, or childhood trauma, or it may be that a major life event in adult life precipitates the hoarding behaviour.
- People with a variety of neurodevelopmental disorders and neurodivergencies may present with hoarding. This could be due to difficulty in sorting and classifying possessions as well as excessive attachment to the stored items.

3

• • • • • • •

Hoarding Disorder

In this chapter, we examine the idea of Hoarding Disorder. This relatively new diagnosis was first described in the American Psychiatric Association's *Diagnostic and Statistical Manual of Mental Disorders*, 5th Edition (DSM-5), which was published in 2013. Hoarding Disorder is used to describe hoarding associated with an extreme attachment to items which are hoarded. Although people with Hoarding Disorder may suffer from other problems such as depression and anxiety, in Hoarding Disorder, it is thought that the hoarding is not due to another diagnosis or problem. However, Hoarding Disorder can present with other diagnoses, as well as with a number of conditions with increased risk taking and impulsivity, and they can be linked, even in the same person, with increased compulsivity and avoidance of risk. Because the concept of Hoarding Disorder has only been described relatively recently, there is a lack of research in this area. Whereas Hoarding Disorder is often described in the elderly or late middle-aged, it is thought to have its roots in childhood. In this chapter, we will examine the presentation of Hoarding Disorder in all age groups.

As well as examining the description and diagnosis of Hoarding Disorder, in this chapter we will also look at the risks inherent in the hoarding itself as well as the risk of suicide. Theories and research about the possible causes of Hoarding Disorder will be discussed.

Treatment of Hoarding Disorder is detailed in later chapters.

What Is Hoarding Disorder and How Is It Distinguished from Hoarding Caused by Another Diagnosis?

Hoarding Disorder is described in the *Diagnostic and Statistical Manual of Mental Disorders*, 5th Edition, Text Revision (DSM-5-TR) as "persistent difficulty in discarding or parting with possessions, regardless of their actual value". In order to make a diagnosis of Hoarding Disorder, the criteria used to make the diagnosis are:

- Difficulty in throwing or giving away items or belongings whether or not they seem valuable to other people.
- The difficulty in throwing away items is linked to the extreme distress and upset that is associated with throwing them away. There is extreme attachment to these belongings.
- This collection of a large number of items due to the difficulty in discarding them causes difficulty in using the living space for its intended use, for example, difficulty cooking in the kitchen due to too many objects, difficulty sleeping in bed due to too many items in bedroom, etc. (if the living areas are not cluttered, it is due to other people clearing up the living areas and not the person who is hoarding the objects).
- The hoarding results in difficulties in social, occupational, or other areas of life, and/or results in significant upset and distress.
- The hoarding is not a result of another medical or mental condition or disorder.

In short, Hoarding Disorder refers to the accumulation of a large number of objects which lead to clutter, and to which the individual has significant emotional attachment, and that this is not better explained by any other medical or mental condition. One of the striking features of Hoarding Disorder is the extreme emotional attachment people with Hoarding Disorder have to their possessions. The tragic story of Penny demonstrates how strong this bond between a person and their hoard can be.

Penny's Story

Penny is a 36-year-old mother of three children aged from 3 to 10 years. Penny had divorced shortly after the birth of her youngest child. She had always had a tendency to hoard items, and this had worsened after the sudden death of her father when she was 12 years old. Living with other people had meant that her hoarding was kept under control to a large extent. Penny particularly liked to hoard items which reminded her of her father. This could include seeing a jumper which was similar to one her father had worn, and she would have an immediate urge to purchase the item. In addition, she kept any items she could which belonged to her father as well as items with his handwriting including simple notes such as shopping lists she had found. Since her husband left the family home 3 years ago, Penny's hoarding had worsened, and she would spend a considerable amount of money on buying men's clothing that she had no intention of wearing but which gave her comfort.

Her ex-husband, George, became very concerned when the children came to stay with him, as they said how nice it was to be able to walk around his house freely whereas it was difficult at home. Further questioning of the children meant that George learned that Penny had now accumulated so many items that she was no longer able to sleep in her bedroom and would sleep in the living room surrounded by piles of clothes and other items. The crowding meant that the television had been moved to the children's bedroom as there was no room in the living room. In addition, the smallest bedroom, which had previously been supposed to be for the oldest child, was so cluttered that all three children were sleeping in the one room. The bathroom was also cluttered, but the bath was still able to be used, and similarly the kitchen was cluttered but usable. George was alarmed and tried to speak with Penny, but she became defensive and refused to let him visit the house, saying she would meet him at the local shopping centre to deliver and collect the children for their weekend visits to their father.

George decided to speak to the school attended by the two eldest children about his concerns. The school confirmed that there had been times they had been worried as the children had arrived in a mixture of odd clothes and not in uniform. When questioned about this they had said that they couldn't find their correct clothes. The school had contacted Penny, but she had claimed that it was because she was having building work and the house was in a mess. As a result of George's and the school's own worries, social services were contacted.

A social worker came to visit Penny when the older children were at school. Penny refused her admission to the house. The social worker spoke to her at the doorstep and became concerned when the youngest child appeared naked despite it being winter and clearly cold in the house. Penny was upset and hostile but eventually agreed that she would be assessed by the local mental health team.

At the appointment with the mental health team, the concerns regarding the children were raised. It was made clear to Penny that it was important that she admit therapists to assess the living situation and also to help her tackle her hoard. Sadly, Penny refused all help. After several months and an emergency trip to the court, Penny lost custody of her children, who were now full time with George, but she could meet them twice a week after school in the shopping centre. When asked about this, it became clear that Penny had such emotional attachment to the items in her hoard that she was willing to sacrifice the close bond she had had with her children. She still deeply loved her children and was distressed at their moving out of the house where she lived, but this was insufficient to motivate her to tackle her Hoarding Disorder. The local mental health team have told her, together with social services, that they are happy to help her whenever she feels able to tackle her hoarding problem.

As mentioned at the start of this book, Hoarding Disorder was only fully described and included as an official diagnosis in DSM-5 in 2013. This relatively recent description of the condition means there is a huge lack of research in Hoarding Disorder. Any research that was performed prior to 2013 is difficult to interpret as it is likely to report on people who may have hoarding as a result of a variety of conditions.

Hoarding Disorder was included in DSM-5 in the section of Obsessive Compulsive and Related Disorders. This means that Hoarding Disorder has many similarities with other conditions in this group and also frequently may present with a combination of these diagnoses. This does not mean that Hoarding Disorder is not found in other conditions – many people with Hoarding Disorder are depressed, for example – but that Hoarding Disorders and other Obsessive Compulsive and Related Disorders are frequently found in the same person or in the family of someone affected. The Obsessive Compulsive and Related Disorders in DSM-5 include:

- F 00 Obsessive Compulsive Disorder
- F 01 Body Dysmorphic Disorder
- F 02 Hoarding Disorder
- F 03 Hair Pulling Disorder (Trichotillomania)
- F 04 Skin Picking Disorder
- F 05–06 Substance-Induced Obsessive Compulsive or Related Disorders
- F 07 Obsessive Compulsive or Related Disorder Associated with a Known General Medical Condition
- F 08 Other Specified Obsessive Compulsive or Related Disorders
- F 09 Unspecified Obsessive Compulsive or Related Disorders

Winston's Story

Winston is a 65-year-old retired train driver who lives alone in a two-bedroom flat in a tower block in the city centre. He had no history of any psychological issues and had always been in good physical health, rarely visiting his general practitioner (GP) and only attending for routine check-up appointments. He had been living with his older brother, Douglas, at the same address since birth in the flat that had belonged to his parents. Winston was born in the UK, but his parents and brother moved to the UK from the Caribbean in the 1950s. The whole family maintained some links with the Caribbean and would often spend holidays there. Douglas decided that he wished to return to the place he was born and bought a house in his birthplace and moved there at the age of 73, 2 years before Winston came to the attention of local authorities.

Winston had always been a quiet man and had very few friends and seemed to have few interests. His job as a train driver meant he spent considerable amounts of time alone. He had rarely socialised with colleagues. The neighbours in his apartment block reported that they rarely saw Winston but that he was always pleasant and polite when they did see him.

At Christmas 2 years after Douglas had left the UK, a fire broke out in the apartment block. Luckily, the alarm was sounded early and the fire brigade attended and everyone escaped without injury. It was apparent that the fire had started in Winston's flat. The officers that attended were extremely concerned by the fact that the flat was filled with papers, magazines, and multiple other items. It appeared that the fire had started as Winston had tried to cook on an open gas flame but the papers piled up around the cooker caught fire, and due to the number of items in the flat, the fire had spread rapidly. It was fortunate that this had occurred during the day as everyone in the apartments was awake and able to respond quickly when the fire alarms sounded.

The flat was uninhabitable but Winston was insistent that he wanted to stay there overnight. It was soaked with water as the fire brigade had put out the flames and in addition was extremely cold and smelt damp as it was apparent that he had not had any heating on for a considerable time as the boiler and radiators were inaccessible due to hoarded materials. The fire brigade and police became concerned and arranged for Winston to have an emergency mental health assessment.

After being taken to the local mental health assessment facility by the police, it was decided that Winston did not have symptoms of depression, psychosis, cognitive impairment, or any other diagnosis. He seemed to have full mental capacity in almost all areas apart from in relation to his flat. Mental capacity means that a person can understand information and make a decision about their life and actions. Assessing mental capacity means assessing an individual's ability to make decisions based on their ability to:

- Understand the situation
- Retain the information

- Weigh up the pros and cons of a decision
- Make a final decision

Winston was alert, bright and quick-witted and was deemed to have full capacity with the exception of his decision to return to his now uninhabitable flat, which was deemed to be unsafe and unhygienic. Winston agreed that the hospital could speak with his brother. Douglas talked to him and eventually agreed that Winston would stay overnight in a local hotel and that his brother would return to the UK as soon as he could arrange a flight. The flat was boarded up so that it was not accessible to intruders.

So that a full survey of the structure of the building could take place, Winston was told that the flat had to be completely cleared. When Douglas arrived, Winston reluctantly agreed for the entire contents of his flat to be packed in boxes and put into a storage facility so that he could sort through them. It soon became apparent that most of the accumulated papers and items were completely useless, having either been burned or destroyed by water as the fire brigade had extinguished the fire. Despite this, Winston became extremely upset and tearful about parting with any of his possessions. Douglas was persistent and eventually some items were placed in boxes in storage, but the rest were in such a state that they were thrown away. As this was going on, Douglas became increasingly worried about his brother's mental state as Winston became even more withdrawn and had lost his appetite and stopped taking any interest in the clearance that was going on. Urged by his brother, he went to see his GP who had known him for many years and realised that he was now severely depressed and suicidal. Winston was admitted to the local mental health hospital for help with his depression and his marked suicidal ideas. Whilst being treated for his depression, Winston was assessed by his local community psychologist, who discussed with him approaching treatment for his Hoarding Disorder. Although highly sceptical, Winston agreed to engage in psychological treatment for his hoarding issues.

Winston's story demonstrates the link between Hoarding Disorder and the risk of depression. But it also raises some other issues concerning risk and hoarding.

What Other Conditions Are Frequently Associated with Hoarding Disorder?

We have already mentioned that Hoarding Disorder is part of a group of conditions known as the Obsessive Compulsive and Related Disorders. People with Hoarding Disorder may frequently also have symptoms of Obsessive Compulsive Disorder (OCD), and this will be discussed in Chapter 5. Many other conditions may also occur along with Hoarding Disorder, and these will be briefly mentioned here, with further details throughout the book.

- **Depression**

Depression is a complication of all of the Obsessive Compulsive and Related Disorders and is so common that it is unusual to see someone with one of these conditions that is not also depressed to some degree. Hoarding Disorder is no exception to this rule. Indeed, people with Hoarding Disorder may even be more prone to depression due to the social isolation and stigma which frequently accompanies this disorder.

- **Anxiety**

Just as depression is very common in people with all Obsessive Compulsive and Related Conditions including Hoarding Disorder, so are anxiety and some of the anxiety disorders.

- **Obsessive Compulsive Disorder**

In Chapter 5, we will look in detail at how some people with OCD may appear to have Hoarding Disorder, but closer examination shows that they have hoarding symptoms as a function of their obsessions and compulsions. In addition, some people with OCD do also have Hoarding Disorder. The treatment is different in each of these cases, and this is why it is discussed fully later in the book.

- **Obsessive Compulsive Personality Disorder**

People with Obsessive Compulsive Personality Disorder often have hoarding symptoms, and indeed these are one of the symptoms which make it possible to make this diagnosis. The overlap between Hoarding Disorder and Obsessive Compulsive Personality Disorder is huge and will be discussed in Chapter 5.

- **Neurodevelopmental Disorders**

People with autism may hoard due to their desire for sameness and dislike of change as well as some of their extreme interests.

Attention Deficit Hyperactivity Disorder (ADHD) is frequently associated with Hoarding Disorder, and indeed some of the newer treatments for Hoarding Disorder have arisen due to their efficacy in ADHD. These conditions will be fully discussed in Chapter 6.

- **Substance Misuse**

In the past, it was often thought that impulsivity was opposite to compulsivity. In reality, they are often linked in the same person. For example, whereas many people with OCD are less likely to smoke or take illicit drugs, a small but substantial proportion do engage in excessive drinking, drug taking, and other "risk-taking behaviours". There is also some evidence that possibly more people with Hoarding Disorder may use either alcohol or drugs to reduce their symptoms or may be more impulsive.

- **Eating Disorders**

Eating disorders may be more impulsive such as Bulimia or more compulsive such as Anorexia Nervosa, and indeed the impulsive vs. compulsive elements are frequently seen in these individuals. People with Hoarding Disorder frequently self-neglect, but in some this may be due to Hoarding Disorder. Some people with eating disorders may also have either autism or another developmental disorder or Obsessive Compulsive Personality Disorder.

As can be seen from the examples above, the overlap between conditions is complex. The issue of impulsivity versus compulsivity is only just being examined and is not fully understood. Figure 3.1 is a diagrammatic representation of the overlap of many disorders and how they differ in their impulsivity/compulsivity/risk-taking features found in any one individual. Of course, this diagram cannot tell the whole truth, but thinking about where a person falls on the risk-taking spectrum may be helpful in planning treatment.

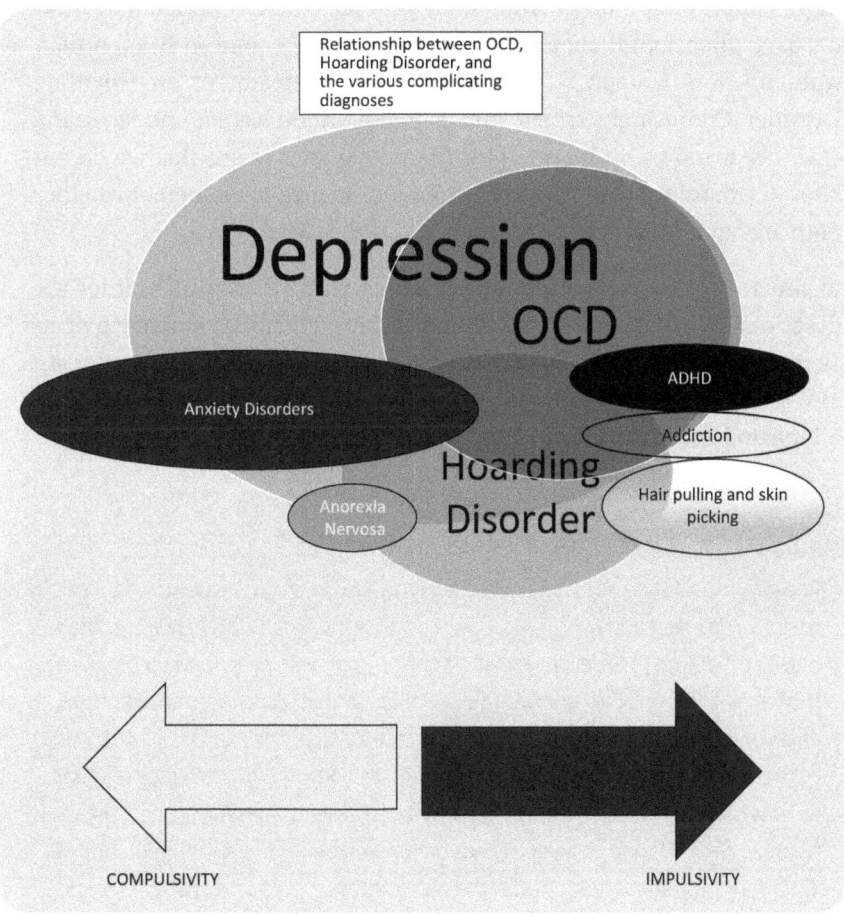

Figure 3.1 Overlap of features.

Who Develops Hoarding Disorder?

Whereas Hoarding Disorder was often thought of as a problem of older-aged adults and the elderly, more recent research has found evidence that it typically starts in childhood or adolescence and can then, untreated, worsen over the individual's life.

There are mixed findings when looking at whether Hoarding Disorder is more common in men or women. In general, whereas population studies have often found Hoarding Disorder is more common in men than women, more women tend to seek help and treatment for Hoarding Disorder. Confusingly, recent studies in childhood have found Hoarding Disorder is more common in girls than boys, so it seems that we do not know if Hoarding Disorder is more frequent in men or women or whether both are equally likely to be affected.

In much of the medical literature, people with Hoarding Disorder are described as being perfectionistic and to have difficulties in making decisions due to this perfectionism. Many people with Hoarding Disorder are also found to be people who tend to procrastinate or in other words to put off making decisions.

Rosemary's Story

Rosemary is a 45-year-old legal secretary who lives in an outer suburb of a small town. Unmarried and with few social contacts, Rosemary had always prided herself on doing an excellent job at work. She had been described by previous bosses as "the perfect employee", being diligent, hard-working, conscientious, and someone who would always stay on late at work to ensure her work was of the highest standard. In the past, her bosses had tried to introduce a junior to Rosemary in order to help her in her work. These appointments had always failed as her juniors found her impossible to work with due to her demands of extremely high standards. Overall, she was found to be a somewhat prickly and difficult person to work with who was as critical of others as she was of herself, and as a result, she had worked alone on specific jobs for the past 15 years.

Six months ago, a neighbour complained to the local council that they were unable to get into the shared driveway to their garage due to the accumulation of a large number of items in boxes which were spilling out from Rosemary's home.

A council official came round to see what was happening and told Rosemary she would have to move these boxes as they were creating a hazard with a risk of someone falling over them. Upon hearing this, Rosemary became very angry and started writing extreme letters to the council alleging they were bullying her. She also began writing abusive and threatening letters to her neighbour. Due to the nature of these letters, the police were informed and visited Rosemary to caution her against such actions. The police became concerned when they visited her property and saw how it appeared that the property was full of hoarded items.

The story of Rosemary describes a middle-aged lady who has few friends and who appears to be "picky" and somewhat perfectionistic. Whereas her striving for perfection at work could be seen as an advantage to the legal firm she worked with, it was difficult for colleagues. Her striving for perfection meant she had difficulty in making up her mind to discard items, and consequently, over the years her home had become increasingly hoarded and difficult for her to live in.

Of course, not everyone with Hoarding Disorder has a similar personality. Many people with Hoarding Disorder do have friends and are close to their relatives. Most will try and avoid meeting people at their homes due to the shame of having a messy home, but many will otherwise socialise and be popular members of their community.

Risks Associated with Hoarding Disorder

It is not surprising that excessive hoarding, particularly the most extreme types seen in Hoarding Disorder, can result in injury and sadly even death in some individuals. Risks include those of fire, but also when items are packed into an area the inhabitants risk injury due to falling, and also from an "avalanche" of possessions under which a person can become trapped.

A famous tragic story of extreme hoarding was that of the Collyer brothers who lived in Harlem in New York from 1885 to 1947 when they died aged 61 years and 65 years. They collected a huge hoard of books, furniture, musical instruments, and a variety of other possessions. While early in life they had gone out to work and mixed with the local community, in middle age they became increasingly isolated and started to live like hermits. This tendency was strengthened as the neighbours began to spread rumours about the brothers. In his 50s one of the brothers, Homer, suffered loss of sight and became blind and was being cared for by his brother, Langley, who would mainly only venture outdoors when it was dark. Homer then became paralysed due to a rheumatic condition. By the early 1930s the brothers' electricity, telephone, gas, and water were switched off due to failure to pay bills. They would heat the home with a small kerosene lamp. There had been a small fire in the property and Langley had refused to let the firemen see or speak with his brother. Over the next few years, Langley fell into more issues with authorities and his failure to pay bills. He accumulated huge piles of newspapers, which he claimed he was keeping so that when Homer regained his sight, he could catch up on the news. In 1947, the police were suspicious and entered the property, digging for 5 hours through possessions until they came across the body of Homer. As Langley was nowhere to be found, it was speculated that he had fled the property. The police continued to clear the flat and, tragically, 18 days after Homer's body had been discovered, Langley was found dead, having been crushed by his possessions.

Although the tragic story of the Collyer brothers in New York was many decades ago, there are still huge risks associated with hoarding. In Chapter 1, we saw that in 2022, the London Fire Brigade attended 1036 hoarding-related fires which resulted in 186 injuries and 10 deaths.[1] In Wales, it was reported that hoarding was responsible for 25–30 per cent of fire-related deaths.[2]

Fires, injuries, and falls are sadly not the only risks from Hoarding Disorder. Other risks to health include:

- Poor nutrition due to inability to cook as a result of limited space in the kitchen.

- Danger of cold and hypothermia due to inability to reach heaters and radiators.
- Damage to health from damp due to cold resulting in mould, etc.
- Unsanitary conditions caused by rotting debris, such as food, can lead to infection and infestations.

As well as the risks of self-neglect in hoarding which may result in conditions such as heart and lung disease and even diabetes due to lack of nutritious food, Hoarding Disorder is often accompanied by other psychiatric conditions such as depression. Later in the book, we will examine how hoarding and Hoarding Disorder interplay with other conditions such as OCD, post-traumatic stress, etc. But depression to some extent is almost universal in hoarding. This is perhaps not surprising. An individual with Hoarding Disorder has a poor quality of life in most cases. Poor physical health is also known to be associated with more depression. In addition to all of these, the stigma surrounding hoarding which results in shame and disgust is also something which feeds the depression. There have been very few studies of suicide in people with Hoarding Disorder, so actual figures may change in future, but it is known that there is a high rate of thoughts of suicide. The reasons for this are likely to be related to the high rate of depression, the social isolation, and the sense of shame experienced by many with Hoarding Disorder. Indeed, studies have suggested that approximately a quarter of people with Hoarding Disorder may attempt to kill themselves over their lifetime.

Hopefully, as the public and professionals learn more about hoarding, this stigma will decrease, but it means that it is vital that someone with Hoarding Disorder is treated with dignity and respect for a problem which they did not choose but which is the result of genetics as well as environment.

Research into the Causes of Hoarding Disorder

The various causes of Hoarding Disorder have not been well researched, due to the relatively recent definition of the condition. However, the general theories of causation can be divided into the following categories:

- Psychological
- Genetic
- Due to the "wiring" of the brain

Of course, none of these three categories excludes any of the others, so it may be that someone has a strong genetic likelihood to develop Hoarding Disorder, which has resulted in a particular way of thinking, resulting in increased likelihood of developing Hoarding Disorder.

Psychological Theories

Many, but not all people who live with Hoarding Disorder, have a history of a deprived or unhappy childhood. This could take the form of living in poverty with few possessions as a child, which can result in retaining all possessions obtained in later life. This can be seen as a reaction to times of scarcity but can take over the person's world when too many items are accumulated. The extreme attachment to the items can also be understood in the case of a person who has had little in early life and may always fear deep down they may return to this lack of belongings. Similarly, some people who grow up in environments with little love and affection may instead form very strong bonds and start to "love" their possessions, even if many of them seem to have little value to the outside world.

Carl's Story

Carl is a 35-year-old man who lives alone in one room in a shared house. The state of the room has caused complaints from his housemates as it is packed with clothes which he mainly buys from charity shops. He started to spill these items out into the communal areas, but his housemates disposed of many of these, which they felt were little more than rags. Carl became very distressed when this happened, and started a fight with the housemate he felt was the main perpetrator. Since that time, he has refused to come out into the communal areas except after dark when the rest of the house is in bed.

In early life, Carl grew up in a traveller community with six brothers and sisters. There was very little money in the household, and Carl always wore clothes that were too small for his older siblings. He rarely attended school and often played truant, but when he did attend, he was bullied and mocked for being "smelly and dirty". He left school at 16, and since then has only had occasional casual labouring and other unskilled work. As soon as he receives money, Carl tends to spend it on new clothes which he buys new from discount stores or second-hand from charity shops. He spends nearly all his money on such purchases and consequently has a very poor diet and is thin and undernourished in appearance. This lack of nutrition has resulted in many physical health problems such as iron deficiency anaemia, folate deficiency anaemia, and other issues.

Carl's story shows how some people who grow up in poverty may develop Hoarding Disorder. The story of Aimee shows how a different type of deprivation may result in similar problems.

Aimee's Story

Aimee is a 25-year-old woman who lives in a luxury apartment in an expensive central city location. Although her living space is a good size, every room is stuffed full of possessions so that she can no longer use her bath and can only sleep on the edge of the bed, which is otherwise piled high with toys, books, and other items.

Born into an extremely wealthy aristocratic family, Aimee rarely spent time with her parents, who tended to be aloof and not be affectionate towards her. Instead, she was raised by a series of paid nannies. Aimee formed strong bonds with many of these nannies but most would only stay for 1–2 years and then Aimee would cry for days when one she had become close to would leave. At the age of 8, she was sent to a boarding school. Unhappy at this school, and unable to make many friends, Aimee became very attached to her soft toys and dolls, which she described as her "friends".

> After leaving school, Aimee worked as a receptionist in a socialite night club. She spent considerable amounts of her salary on toys. Initially, this seemed controllable, but over the years, it became completely out of hand until her flat was crammed with items. When asked if she would sort her toys, Aimee was tearful and exclaimed that she loved each and every one and that they were her only "friends".

Not all people with Hoarding Disorder have histories of deprivation such as Carl and Aimee. There have been many suggestions as to which factors may make this type of extreme attachment to objects more likely. These factors, such as difficulty in categorising items, will be discussed under other headings below. Once an attachment to the items has developed, then the avoidance of throwing away items strengthens the belief that discarding items would be distressing and painful.

Genetic Families and How Hoarding Disorder Can Run in Families

There is good evidence that Hoarding Disorder runs in families. Just because a certain condition runs in families does not necessarily mean it is down to genes and genetics. A high proportion of older adults who have Hoarding Disorder report that their mothers also hoarded when they were growing up. Therefore, it could be the environment they grew up in which resulted in the Hoarding Disorder, or it could be due to genes which made it more likely. One of the ways that researchers try to distinguish between the effects of genes and the environments is to study identical and non-identical twins.

Identical twins share all the same genes whereas non-identical twins share half their genes, as do non-twin siblings. It has been found that identical twins who have a twin with Hoarding Disorder are considerably more likely to develop Hoarding Disorder than non-identical twins, even though they have shared the same environment. This does not mean that, if an identical twin does have Hoarding Disorder, it is inevitable that the other will develop it, but that it is more likely than for the general population.

Brain Wiring and Hoarding Disorder

All of us process and retain information in different ways. For example, at school some children find arithmetic easy, whereas others may struggle with arithmetic but be excellent at other subjects such as English. Similarly, the way our brains deal with and sort information can vary.

Many people with Hoarding Disorder have some differences in how they process and sort information. There are relatively few studies in this area and, as already mentioned, many people with Hoarding Disorder have not sought treatment or have not been diagnosed. However, it does seem that many people with Hoarding Disorder have difficulties in the following areas:

- Sorting and categorising items
- Attention
- Decision making

In order to decide what items need to be kept and stored, thrown away or given to others, it is necessary to be able to categorise and sort items. Some people find this more difficult than others. This categorisation can be a problem for people with Hoarding Disorder.

Adam's Story

Adam is a 40-year-old man who works in a hospital as a porter. He lives in a house with his wife, but she complains about his disorganisation. Recently, she discovered that Adam had been keeping dishes in a cupboard in the bathroom as well as in the bedroom wardrobe. When asked about this, Adam did not feel this was a problem even though they now had accumulated a huge number of dishes.

Adam demonstrates a difficulty in being able to categorise items correctly. Similarly people may have difficulty in distinguishing between items of high and low value, for example, broken crockery, as opposed to functional cups and saucers.

Another common problem is that many people with Hoarding Disorder have difficulty in maintaining their attention. For example, someone with an inability to pay attention for any length of time will find it difficult to categorise, decide on what to do with the item, and then dispose of the unnecessary items.

Faye's Story

Faye is a 50-year-old woman who lives with her husband and two teenaged daughters in a farmhouse in a rural part of the UK. She has always been described as a little "hare-brained" and did poorly at school due to constant daydreaming. Once she set up home with her husband after moving from her parents' family home, it became clear that Faye was disorganised and chaotic. The house the family lives in has always been kept tidy by her husband. If left to her own devices, Faye would leave items all over the house and would not clear up after herself. Although these difficulties caused arguments initially, her family all help in the house whilst Faye takes on tasks which do not demand high concentration.

As well as ability to categorise and to pay attention, the last ability people need to have to avoid hoarding is the ability to make decisions. It has been noted that many people with Hoarding Disorder are undecided and spend much longer making decisions in many areas of life compared to many people without Hoarding Disorder.

Gender and Hoarding Disorder

The issue of whether more men or women have Hoarding Disorder is one which is not really known. Some researchers have suggested that Hoarding Disorder is more common in men rather than women whereas some recent studies have suggested that more women are in treatment for Hoarding Disorder, and that more women report severe Hoarding Disorder. It is difficult to know what this means. It is possible that women are more likely to recognise they have a problem and to seek treatment, or it could be that as Hoarding Disorder is often not recognised until older age, more women live long enough for this problem to become apparent. In short, we need many more studies to examine if there are any differences in frequency of Hoarding Disorder in men and women.

When we look at the distressing issue of Animal Hoarding, it is known that this is more common in women than in men. This type of hoarding in discussed fully in Chapter 4.

Hoarding Disorder in Children and Adolescents

It was often thought that Hoarding Disorder was a condition of older adults, as this is the time when it is most frequently seen in clinical practice. We have already discussed how this may be related to the fact that people are more likely to live alone as they age, and that living with someone else who intervenes and prevents hoarding from getting out of hand seems to be a protective factor. However, studies on older people with Hoarding Disorder have generally found that many of them report their issues as starting from childhood.

Hoarding in childhood may easily be overlooked as parents may prevent the hoard getting out of hand, the child does not generally have access to much space beyond their bedrooms or other areas in the house, and they will have less purchasing power. Nevertheless, there are now many reports on children and adolescents with Hoarding Disorder.

We have already commented on the lack of studies of Hoarding Disorder in general, and this lack is even more marked in the case of young people. Preliminary studies in a number of Western countries seem to suggest that almost 1 per cent of children may have some difficulties with hoarding. Some researchers have reported that Hoarding Disorder may be more frequent in girls rather than boys. Unsurprisingly, it is often found that a parent or close relative may also have symptoms of Hoarding Disorder. It has also been suggested that almost half of those with hoarding may also have another psychological issue such as anxiety or depression, as well as some with neurodevelopmental issues such as ADHD or autism. In terms of age at onset of hoarding problems, it seems most are around the age of puberty with a few starting at a younger age.

Children will hoard for similar reasons to adults. It has already been noted that adolescents are often untidy and may appear to hoard items, but they will differ from someone with Hoarding Disorder in the amount of emotion that they feel towards the hoarding objects. Of course, children and adolescents may all feel close emotional bonds with items which are of little value to others, such as the much-loved but barely recognisable stuffed toy, or the scruffy jacket beloved by an adolescent, but generally they may not have such strong feelings about the items which are piling up on their bedroom floor and will be relatively happy if a parent cleans up the space for them. A child with Hoarding Disorder, however, will actively mourn the loss of any of their hoarded items.

Phoebe's Story

Phoebe is an 11-year-old girl who lives with her mother in a large city. Her father left the family home when she was 2 years old, but he maintains weekly visits where he takes Phoebe on an outing to a local park, to the cinema, or sometimes for a meal. Phoebe's mother, Caroline, became concerned as Phoebe had started collecting a large number of items which she was attempting to hide at the back of the cupboard. When Caroline examined these, they consisted of a large number of stones, twigs, a pizza box, and general items she had collected whilst out with her father. When Caroline said to Phoebe that these items would need to be thrown away as they were becoming smelly and a risk of attracting vermin, Phoebe became distraught. She said she loved these items and that she could not bear to part with them. Caroline was surprised by the vehemence and extreme emotion that Phoebe was showing so suggested they went through the items together. Phoebe reluctantly agreed to this. It was suggested by Caroline that she could keep the stones and the twigs, leaves, and pieces of paper, but that items which were covered in food, such as pizza boxes, needed to be thrown away. Hearing that anything was to be thrown away led to Phoebe throwing herself on the ground and pleading with her mother. Caroline decided to leave it at present and to go back when Phoebe was at school to clear the items that were a risk of vermin, believing Phoebe might not notice.

The next day Caroline searched through the pile and found six pizza boxes along with multiple food wrappers and foil. She placed these in the rubbish bin. When Phoebe came home, she went to her bedroom and then began shouting and wailing, accusing her mother of "taking away my best friends". At first, Caroline did not realise that by talking of her "best friends" Phoebe was referring to the items she had thrown out. The level of Phoebe's distress was such that Caroline agreed to retrieve the items from the bin on condition that they went and discussed it with the GP the next day.

Phoebe reluctantly agreed to see the doctor with her mother on condition her mother would not discard her items but would store them in the garage. The GP made a referral to the local child and adolescent mental health team, where Phoebe was diagnosed and underwent treatment for her Hoarding Disorder, as well as family meetings with her father and mother. At one of these meetings, it was revealed that one of the reasons why Phoebe's parents had divorced was due to her father's hoarding behaviour.

Occasionally younger children will exhibit signs and symptoms of Hoarding Disorder. Not all children have a clear family history of Hoarding Disorder, nor do they always have evidence of any emotional trauma at all.

Ruaridh's Story

Ruaridh is an 8-year-old boy who lives with his parents in a cosy suburban house close to his maternal grandparents. He is a bright child who does well at school and who loves to make things. Recently, his mother moved the sofa to find 10 toilet roll tubes hidden behind it. On asking Ruaridh if these were his, he explained they were and that he was collecting them to "make things". At first his mother didn't take much notice but then discovered that Ruaridh had been collecting and hiding toilet roll and kitchen roll tubes all over the house and even had hidden some at his grandparents' house. On final counting, it was discovered that he had accumulated in the region of 100 cardboard tubes from his parents' and grandparents' houses and from school. His parents told him that this was far too many and he couldn't possibly be planning to use all of them, but Ruaridh was insistent and threw a tantrum at the idea of disposing of any of these.

His mother, Mary, went to see his teacher to ask if there were any projects which required cardboard tubes. The teacher confirmed that there were no such projects. She said, however, that she was pleased with Ruaridh's academic progress and was not concerned about him unduly. She did say he seemed to be quite a shy and withdrawn child who did not mix much with the other children, and asked if anything was happening at home which might be stressful. Mary said that there was nothing she could think of.

Mary went home feeling very guilty and wondering if anything she or the family had done had led to Ruaridh's behaviour. The next day she made an appointment to see her GP. The GP had known Mary for several years and was surprised how distressed she was. He reassured her that he was sure there was nothing she could have done to prevent this behaviour and arranged for Ruaridh to be seen by local child and adolescent mental health services.

Ruaridh did well in treatment and does seem happier. His mother was delighted when he decided to invite two schoolfriends home to play as this was something he had not previously done himself.

Ruaridh's story illustrates the very important point that, although parents will nearly always blame themselves for any issues experienced by their children, this is not helpful or true. The vast majority of parents are trying their best to give their children what they need given the circumstances they find themselves in. Most psychological problems in their children are unrelated to their behaviour. These conditions tend to run in families and be due to genetic factors, or they may be caused by the socioeconomic situation the family finds themselves in. Parent blaming is an unhelpful and untrue action!

KEY POINTS

- Hoarding Disorder refers to a condition which was only described as a diagnosis in 2013 and which is one of the conditions described as Obsessive Compulsive and Related Disorders (OCaRDs).

- Hoarding Disorder can occur alongside Obsessive Compulsive Disorder or the other OCaRDs but is a standalone condition in its own right.

- Hoarding Disorder can also be complicated by other diagnoses including other OCaRDs, depression, anxiety, neurodevelopmental, and conditions related to increased impulsivity and risk taking.

- Compulsivity and Impulsivity appear at first sight to be opposites, but in reality, they often overlap even in the same individual.

- Hoarding Disorder can present at any age, but recent research suggests it may frequently start in childhood and only be recognised later in life.

- It used to be thought that Hoarding Disorder was more common in men, but studies have mixed findings. Recent studies seem to suggest that women are more likely to seek or be referred for treatment for Hoarding Disorder.

- Hoarding Disorder presents a number of risks to the individual and also to neighbours from hazards such as:
  - Fire
  - Structural damage to properties
  - Crushing of individuals due to an "avalanche" of items
  - Infection and infestation in the hoard

- There is a high rate of suicidal behaviour in people with Hoarding Disorder, and it is often accompanied by depression and anxiety.

- Social stigma worsens the situation in Hoarding Disorder.

- Hoarding Disorder often runs in families and seems to have a genetic basis.

- Some people with Hoarding Disorder have a history of childhood poverty or lack of love in early childhood, and sometimes these factors may result in excessive attachment to objects.
- Difficulties in performing certain tasks relating to classification and sorting of items and in attention have been found in some people with Hoarding Disorder.

4

• • • • • • •

Animal Hoarding

In this chapter, we will examine the condition of Animal Hoarding. The various types of people who may hoard more animals than they are able to care for will be examined. Although some animal hoarders frequently also hoard inanimate objects as well, there are some differences in those who hoard animals and inanimate objects. These differences will be presented and discussed. Socioeconomic factors play a part in people who actively hoard animals, as well as those who inadvertently find themselves overwhelmed by the number of their animals. The management and treatment of Animal Hoarding is less researched than the hoarding of other items, and this will be mentioned along with descriptions of the treatments which may be helpful.

Introduction

We have already seen that Hoarding Disorder was not recognised as a condition separate from Obsessive Compulsive Disorder (OCD) and Obsessive Compulsive Personality Disorder (OCPD) until it was described in 2013. Animal Hoarding has been even less researched and has often been dealt with at a later stage by the animal rescue agencies, veterinarians, housing officers, environmental officers, and ultimately the law.

Animal Hoarding may be described as the accumulation of a larger number of animals than the individual can afford to care for or is physically able to look after. As a result, animals are neglected and ultimately sick, dying, or dead when help is obtained. According to the animal welfare agencies, there are three main types of people who have large numbers of animals.

- Firstly, there are people who have a more typical Hoarding Disorder but have large collections of animals which they are unable to care for properly. Some of these people will also hoard other items as well as animals. The rest of this chapter will concentrate on this group and the similarities and differences to hoarding only of possessions.

- Secondly, there are people who are animal lovers and have several pets. Sometimes due to unplanned breeding they may be in a position where they may have more animals than they can cope with. Alternatively, they may have been able to look after their animals for many years but then an alteration in their financial situation, such as the loss of a job, or a deterioration in their physical or mental health, may make them unable to properly care for the animals themselves. These people do not usually have Hoarding Disorder as we have described it. Indeed, many such people may approach animal welfare agencies for help or may be heartbroken but surrender their animals for adoption. However, others may be too ashamed or too attached to their animals to consider such an option. Other mental health issues may also compound these problems. These will be discussed in this chapter, as it is often difficult to distinguish these people from the true hoarders. For the purposes of this chapter, we will refer to these people as Overwhelmed Carers.

- Finally, there are unscrupulous people who are looking to gain financially from the animals. These are exploitative people with no care about the animals or the suffering of animals. These people are not classified as animal hoarders but as criminal traders. These only make up approximately 10 per cent of animal cruelty cases with large numbers of animals. However, these are breeders and "puppy farmers" and many may go undetected. These people will not be discussed further in this chapter.

As well as Animal Hoarding, there are other diagnoses that may result in animal hoarding behaviours. People with Bipolar Disorder may acquire larger numbers of animals than they can realistically look after during a "high" but in this case, reason will normally mean they can work to reduce the issue once they have a stable mood. Other conditions which may result in Animal Hoarding are dementia and psychotic illnesses. These conditions could also complicate and exist alongside Animal Hoarding.

Animal Hoarding

The most common animals that are hoarded are cats and dogs, but rabbits, guinea pigs, birds, and other small animals may also be hoarded. More women than men hoard animals, and it is most commonly seen in middle-aged unmarried women, and is more common in those who live alone. When men hoard animals, they have a greater tendency to hoard dogs, while women have a slightly greater tendency to hoard cats.

In hoarded homes, the person collects large numbers of animals. This increase in numbers may arise through unplanned breeding but is often also due to the individual deciding to "rescue" the animals. In addition, once it is known in a locality that this person "rescues" animals, other people may drop off animals with a view to them being rehomed. Sometimes they may set up small unregulated animal "charities" and promote that they rehome animals. Being hugely bonded and emotionally attached to these animals, the hoarder can rarely bear to part with any of them, even to obviously good homes. Due to the number of animals and the overwhelming nature of the task, the home becomes overrun with animals that the individual is unable to care for. The home environment becomes squalid, and often animal urine and faeces are found throughout the living areas. This is unsatisfactory for both the humans and the animals. Unhygienic conditions can often lead to increased illnesses amongst the animals, and living in very close quarters in unsanitary conditions further increases rates of illness. The person with the hoarding problem may resist seeking veterinary help for sick animals due to financial worries, fear that the veterinarian may report them to animal welfare authorities, or because they are in self-denial of their state of affairs.

The overwhelming emotion the individual feels is extreme love for the animals, and many people may believe they are the only person that could ever love their animals as much. This belief and passionate love is one reason why the animals aren't voluntarily rehomed elsewhere even if potential adoptees come forward. Clearly this leads to a tragic situation for both the animals and the humans involved. Reports have shown that in 60 per cent of animal hoarded homes, dead animals are found as well as extremely sick animals, when the authorities have intervened. The smell and noise from the animals, and general concern from neighbours means that people who hoard animals are likely to be referred to local authorities or animal welfare agencies. A multi-agency approach usually follows, with attempts to improve the living situation of both the animals and the humans. Even after animals are removed or helped, there is a high risk that a similar situation will recur once the agencies cease their involvement.

This is a very sad situation in many cases. People with Animal Hoarding often lack insight, deny there is a problem, and refuse help. Unfortunately, this results in the courts being the end result in many of these situations. This is also unhelpful in the long term as the individual who is hoarding animals feels persecuted and wronged.

We have already looked at the shame and reluctance to admit to a problem in people with Hoarding Disorder. This is even more profound in Animal Hoarding as people are shocked and appalled by the animal suffering. In addition, the fact that these people are often not seen as having a mental health problem but are viewed as people who need to be dealt with by the courts adds to the stigma, shame, and resentment of society felt by the person who is hoarding.

With the recognition of Hoarding Disorder as a mental condition in its own right, mental health services are increasingly becoming involved in offering help and treatment to people with hoarding issues. Animal Hoarding is less well understood, but with the development of more hoarding services, it is hoped more treatment will be offered in the future.

Olga's Story

Olga is a 53-year-old unmarried lady who lives in a small two-bedroomed flat with a small outside balcony in London. Never having married or had close friends, Olga had moved to the UK aged 25 years to escape poverty in her homeland. She initially worked as a translator for a large firm of international lawyers, having learnt English in her school. At work, Olga was an efficient member of staff but never joined in any of the social life; she always liked to get away on time to get home to her cats. After 5 years with the firm, Olga left to become a freelance interpreter.

It became well known in her neighbourhood that Olga would take in any stray or abandoned cats. She advertised in the local shops as "Olga's Cat Rescue". In recent years, her neighbours began complaining about a strong smell coming from her flat. Initially they asked her if she could stop putting out used cat litter and items on her balcony. Olga became immediately defensive on the suggestion of any smell, but did move some items from her balcony. The smell remained but when the neighbours approached Olga again, she became verbally abusive and accused them of bullying her and threatened to report them to the police.

A neighbourhood community group operated in her block of flats and was comprised of people who lived in the flats, whether owner-occupiers or renters. Their meetings were well attended although Olga had never done so. The issue with the smell emanating from Olga's flat was discussed at a meeting. After discussion, it was decided that the best course of action would be for the chairperson to write a friendly letter to Olga explaining the issue that they were having with the smell. Unfortunately, this seemed to escalate matters further. Neighbours began to receive anonymous offensive letters that they believed came from Olga. One of the group suggested that the Royal Society for the Prevention of Cruelty to Animals (RSPCA) should be contacted as they began to be concerned about the wellbeing of her cats.

At first, the RSPCA wanted to ensure that this was not a malicious accusation on behalf of the neighbours. They wrote to Olga and asked if they could speak with her. Olga wrote back a venomous reply saying that she knew they were all scoundrels who wanted to harm her and her animals. The RSPCA wrote again and explained they wanted to help her and her animals, and that if her animals were fine and healthy, no further steps would be taken. However, because their investigations had now led them to believe that the animals might be at risk, they were visiting again and would obtain a warrant to enter her property if she was non-compliant. When the RSPCA officers arrived at her property, Olga refused them entry, screaming at them through the letterbox and refusing to open the door. She threatened that, if they did not leave, she would beat them with an iron bar which she claimed to have at the ready. The officers tried to reason with her but to no avail.

The RSPCA then applied for a warrant to enter Olga's property and asked for police assistance as they were anxious about her threats of violence towards them.

When they returned to Olga's flat with the police, Olga still resisted opening the door but, on seeing the police were there, eventually opened the door. Once they got inside the flat, they saw rooms which seemed to be covered with cats and smelled strongly of urine and excrement. It was obvious that there was excrement in several places on the floor. The bedroom, bathroom, and kitchen were all as filthy as the main room and hallway. The RSPCA found there were 60 cats all in a state of malnutrition and many looking extremely sickly and unwell. Further investigation found three dead cats in the freezer which Olga said were there because she had not had time to find a place to bury them. As well as the cats being undernourished, Olga herself was in a poor state of health, extremely thin, pale, and looking much older than her 53 years. It was agreed with the police and the RSPCA that this situation could not be allowed to continue any longer and that backup should be called to arrange to remove the cats immediately for veterinary care. Olga was by this time weeping and pleading with them not to remove her "babies". Everyone felt extremely concerned about Olga, and the police asked her to go with them to the hospital for a mental health assessment as they believed she was in need of help. Although she did not want to do this, and was insistent there was nothing wrong with her or her animals, she reluctantly agreed as the police told her that they could force her to do this as they were concerned about her wellbeing.

After being taken to the local hospital for mental health assessment, it was agreed that she should be able to go home. The RSPCA had explained to her that they would be back the next day to help her to clear up the mess and to make her flat hygienic for the return of some of her cats. Olga returned home, and with the help of the RSPCA, the flat was completely cleaned and sanitised. Many of her cats were found to be severely undernourished, and two were in such a poor state that they had to be euthanised. With working with Olga, although she refused to accept that her cats were at risk, the RSPCA officers were able to establish a rapport. They eventually agreed that three of her cats could return home. Extremely reluctantly and with many tears, Olga agreed to give up the remaining cats for rehoming. She is attending weekly sessions with a therapist for Cognitive Behaviour Therapy (CBT). Progress has been slow, but there are some small changes in her views even though she feels removal of the animals was unnecessary. She has also been taking an antidepressant, venlafaxine, which has improved her mood and which may have had some effect on her hoarding behaviours.

The story of Olga demonstrates a lady who truly loves her animals but yet sadly ends up in a situation where she is causing her much-loved pets harm. It is particularly tragic that it took so long until her hoarding problems were discovered and dealt with. Earlier intervention could have prevented considerable animal and human suffering. Olga did not demonstrate other hoarding tendencies apart from her cats, but the story of Shelley is different.

Shelley's Story

Shelley is a 26-year-old single-parent mother of two children aged 5 years and 9 years. Both children attend the local primary school. The headteacher became concerned about the older child, a boy called Waylen, who was frequently dishevelled and would fall asleep in class. The younger child Tabitha was less tired but often also dishevelled. When she spoke to Waylen, he said that he wasn't sleeping as he didn't have much room in the bed. On closer questioning, the headteacher discovered that Waylen, Tabitha, his mother, and several household pets were all sleeping on one bed. The headteacher became concerned and asked to speak with Shelley.

When Shelley was asked about their living situation, she stated that it was fine. Asked if the children had their own bedroom, she insisted that they did. When told what Waylen had said, Shelley denied this was true and said the children had a lovely bedroom with everything they could wish for. The headteacher remained worried, however, and asked local social services to investigate.

When social services contacted Shelley and a social worker, Sharon, said she wanted to visit the house, Shelley kept insisting that she would attend with the children at the social services offices. Wishing to establish a rapport with the family, Sharon agreed to a first meeting there.

Shelley's parents had been poor. She had few possessions and also saw little of her own parents, who were working extremely hard. As a consequence, Shelley was cared for by a variety of neighbours, friends, and acquaintances. She vowed from an early age that her children would not have a similar experience. She fell pregnant at the age of 16, and after being disowned by her parents, moved to bed and breakfast accommodation where she remained until she fell pregnant again and was able to move into a housing association flat. Although she warmed to Sharon, Shelley was extremely reluctant to let her visit at home. Interviewing Waylen and Tabitha on their own without their mother, Sharon became concerned about their stories of all sleeping in one bed and having no room to play. Sharon insisted that she visit the flat and made an appointment for the following week.

On arrival at the flat, it was apparent that Shelley had been tidying as there were several boxes of items in the hallway. Shelley answered the door, and Sharon was taken into the living area. This was covered with toys and very untidy, but she was able to sit down. Sharon knew that Shelley had had permission to keep a dog but was surprised that this was not obvious. They had a cup of tea and talked about how Shelley was coping, and then Sharon asked to look around. Shelley made excuses and tried to dissuade her from doing this. Sharon was insistent and was first shown the children's bedroom. It became immediately clear that there was no space for the children to play or sleep in this room which was piled high with a huge collection of children's toys, many of which appeared broken. Shelley explained she could not resist buying toys that she saw in charity shops or car boot sales. The bathroom was also full of toys, but there was just enough room to enable the children to be bathed. Shelley's bedroom, where the whole family slept, was covered in toys and clothes so that there was only half of a double bed which was available to sleep on. Sharon was even more surprised when she opened the kitchen door and saw a very cluttered area and six small dogs. The dogs appeared thin and seemed to have matted hair. Sharon expressed surprise to see them in this small space and also the number of them. Shelley said that they were her pride and joy along with her children and everyone was very happy living as they did.

After a long discussion, Sharon made it clear to Shelley that she felt the living situation was unsuitable for the children as they did not have space to play, sleep, or keep the things that really mattered to them. She also said she felt that there were too many dogs in a small space and would like the RSPCA to advise and to look at them.

Shelley was embarrassed and upset but agreed to work with Sharon and a member of the community mental health team to help her with her hoarding problems. Over the next few months, Shelley began seeing a therapist and also working with a "befriender" attached to the community mental health team who helped Shelley as she started to sort out her belongings. The RSPCA visited and, although underweight and not having enough space, the dogs were healthy. Over the next few months, the RSPCA also worked with Shelley, who eventually tearfully agreed for four of the dogs to be rehomed.

Now after 9 months of intervention, Shelley's house is clear and the children have a bedroom they can sleep in. There are two dogs and Shelley continues to keep in touch with the RSPCA inspector that helped her. The children are more settled and appear less tired and dishevelled.

There is also a socioeconomic issue with Animal Hoarding. If you have plenty of money and a large house, it is likely to take longer before you are overwhelmed. Indeed, there have been several very wealthy individuals who have collected hundreds of animals but their wealth enables them to keep their animals in a healthy and safe environment. How these situations relate to the squalor and disease-ridden houses of those with less favourable financial circumstances has not been explored.

Animal Hoarding has also been reported as mostly being in urban areas. This is difficult to understand, and it may be that urban Animal Hoarding is more likely to come to the attention of others due to the proximity of others, whereas in rural settings it may be easier for it to go unnoticed.

Treatment of Animal Hoarding

As already discussed, people with animal hoarding issues are often reluctant to come forward for treatment and often deny there is a problem. With increased public awareness and more open discussion of the issues, it is to be hoped that this reluctance may reduce in the future.

An ideal approach to this issue would be a multi-agency approach whereby the animals are helped in collaboration with the hoarder and mental health services are offered to help the hoarding issue. Overall, CBT (as described in Chapter 8) reduces symptoms by a quarter on average.[1]

Medication may also ease the symptoms and suffering of people with Animal Hoarding, and this is discussed in Chapter 7.

Overwhelmed Carers of Animals

The numbers of pets being surrendered to animal charities increases with any increase in the cost of living. For example, with rapidly increasing inflation, animal rescue centres in Scotland (UK) reported an increase of 25 per cent of animals being brought in for rehoming in the first 6 months of 2023 compared to the previous year.[2]

The story of Brian illustrates this kind of problem and demonstrates why it is not a true Hoarding Disorder.

Brian's Story

Brian is a 79-year-old man who lives alone in a small bungalow at the seaside. His wife died from breast cancer 20 years ago, and his children live overseas. Always having been a dog lover, once he retired from his job as a postman, Brian got two dogs from a local rescue centre. After a few years, he was asked to care for another dog by an elderly neighbour who was going into hospital. Happy to help out, Brian took in the dog but sadly his neighbour died. What

Brian only then realised was that this dog was pregnant. It was assumed that the neighbour, who had not had her dog spayed, was unaware of this situation. The result was six puppies. No one Brian knew could take the puppies and, worried for their welfare, he struggled on with nine dogs in a small living space. For a few years, Brian coped well but he then was pulled over while out walking the dogs, which resulted in a painful hip injury. Hospital X-rays revealed he had not fractured any bones, but he was advised to rest and not do much walking for a few weeks. During this time, the magnitude of having nine dogs enclosed in a small house, and being unable to take them on long walks, began to dawn on Brian. It also led him to thinking about what would happen if he were to be taken really ill and had to spend time in hospital himself, or what would happen when he died.

After much soul-searching, Brian contacted a national dog rescue charity. They visited Brian and were surprised by the mess in the house. On discussion with him, it was agreed that he would keep his two original dogs and the dog he inherited from the neighbour but that the other younger dogs would be given for rehoming.

Several months on, Brian is now able to walk, and with three older dogs is less likely to be pulled over. The younger dogs had no problems finding homes and Brian does see some of them regularly when out on walks as they have been rehomed in his home town.

Despite having accumulated a large number of dogs, Brian does not have a hoarding problem. Other issues which have recently caused people to be unable to care for their pets include inflation and the inability to pay for pet food and veterinary care.

KEY POINTS

- Animal Hoarding has been less well researched than other hoarding disorders.

- Most people with Animal Hoarding are seen by animal rescue charities and veterinarians as well as housing officers and local authority environmental officers.

- There may be other diagnoses which result in the accumulation of more animals than the person can care for, including Bipolar Disorder, dementia, and psychosis.

- Animal Hoarding is hugely stigmatised, and this may not be helped by most people being dealt with via the legal system.

- People with Animal Hoarding typically really love and care for their animals and do not realise or have insight into the suffering they cause their pets.

- Whilst many people just hoard animals, others may hoard animals as well as other items.

- Treatment with either individual or group CBT can be useful.

- Medication such as venlafaxine may be helpful.

5

. . . .

Obsessive Compulsive Disorder, Obsessive Compulsive Personality Disorder, Hoarding Disorder, and How They Interact

In this chapter, we will examine how Obsessive Compulsive Disorder (OCD) or Obsessive Compulsive Personality Disorder (OCPD) may interact with Hoarding Disorder. It has already been noted that, prior to 2013, when a separate diagnosis of Hoarding Disorder was described in the *Diagnostic and Statistical Manual of Mental Disorders, 5th Edition, Text Revision (DSM-5-TR)*[1] under the new category of Obsessive Compulsive and Related Disorders, people with Hoarding Disorder were diagnosed as either having OCD or OCPD. In reality, whereas Hoarding Disorder and symptoms of hoarding are common in both OCD and OCPD, not everyone who has Hoarding Disorder also has one of these conditions. On the other hand, hoarding symptoms may be present in both OCD and OCPD without displaying all of the characteristics of Hoarding Disorder. These distinctions can have an effect on what treatments may work for the individual.

Obsessive Compulsive Disorder and Hoarding

It has been shown that approximately 20 per cent of people with Hoarding Disorder also have symptoms of OCD. These people may also have higher levels of anxiety and depression than those without OCD. On the other hand, about 10–15 per cent of people with OCD have symptoms of hoarding which may or may not amount to a full Hoarding Disorder. The story of Glen illustrates someone with OCD who does not have Hoarding Disorder but has hoarding symptoms.

Glen's Story

Glen is a 58-year-old man who has a history of more than 40 years of OCD symptoms. He has always been reluctant to seek treatment but following the death of his wife of 35 years, his children became worried about him storing more and more items in his house, which had become cluttered and unhygienic. They eventually persuaded him to consult with his doctor.

Glen had always been meticulous and fussy even as a child, but following the start of the AIDS epidemic in the early 1980s, he became scared that he might pass on HIV and AIDS to other people. This symptom waxed and waned over the years. Although Glen had never engaged in any activity which was likely to result in infection, he worried that he might have picked it up from using public toilets or by touching something that was "contaminated". Examples of things which Glen thought were "contaminated" included any red marks (which he worried could be blood from someone who was HIV positive), using public toilets, and touching door handles. He would always carry alcohol cleaning gel and clean his hands on multiple occasions. If he felt his clothes had been in contact with "contaminants", he would strip at home and then shower for up to an hour to ensure he was clean. He would never throw any rubbish away without repeatedly washing it until he was convinced that he would not pass on any "HIV contamination". For this reason, throughout their married life, Glen's wife had always dealt with household chores involving the rubbish. Realistically, Glen knew he did not have HIV, but when he had the thoughts that he might spread the "contamination" he could not think rationally and completely believed his obsessive thoughts.

Following the death of his wife, Glen's symptoms worsened but, additionally, because his wife no longer was there to deal with the rubbish accumulating in the house, the house became hoarded, cluttered, smelly, and unhygienic.

His doctor suggested that he should attend the Psychological Therapy in Primary Care service for some graded exposure with self-imposed Exposure and Response Prevention (ERP), which is the type of psychological treatment which is most useful for OCD. This would involve facing up to his fear of catching and passing on HIV in a graded way without performing any of his anxiety-reducing compulsions of excessive Prevention cleaning, washing, and checking. Glen did not feel ready for this step, so his doctor prescribed sertraline, a medication which has a specific effect on obsessions and compulsions as well as treating depression and is one drug of the class known as selective serotonin reuptake inhibitors (SSRIs). In order to reduce the risk of side effects, Glen was started on 50 mg of sertraline every morning for a week and this increased by 50 mg every week until he was on the dose which is known to be the most effective for OCD of 200 mg a day. Glen did have some side effects of slight nausea and headache, but these went away after a few days. Initially, Glen was disappointed as his symptoms did not improve, but his doctor encouraged him to stay on this medication as it usually takes several weeks at the higher dosage for benefits to be seen. After 8 weeks, Glen noticed his fears were reducing. He then felt able to tackle his remaining worries with ERP.

Glen's story illustrates how OCD symptoms themselves can lead to hoarding. However, it is clear that Glen does not have Hoarding Disorder, as he has no attachment to the hoarded objects and only collects them due to his fear of passing on illness to others, and not because he is attached to them. It is obvious that he does have some of the symptoms of Hoarding Disorder such as embarrassment about his situation, isolation, loneliness, and depression, but these can also be symptoms of OCD.

Glen has OCD with fear of contamination, which is a common feature of OCD. Hoarding symptoms that do not comprise Hoarding Disorder are not confined to contamination fears. The example of Anusha may help to demonstrate this.

Anusha's Story

Anusha is a 25-year-old single woman who works as a freelance photographer. Her parents live in another city, but until recently Anusha lived with her grandmother. Two years ago, her grandmother died. Anusha was very distressed and felt she now had no support. She became miserable and depressed and was given antidepressant medication by her doctor. Although this improved her overall mood, Anusha began to exhibit the symptoms of OCD. She had recurrent intrusive thoughts that she would lose something important and that this would result in a serious problem for her. Whenever she went out, she found it difficult to leave her seat for fear she may have dropped something. This caused her to miss her stop on buses and trains and started making it more difficult for her to work. At home, she had increasing issues with disposing of items, and her rubbish accumulated as she felt the need to repeatedly check that she was not discarding something which was important. This problem developed further, and she began to be fearful that she could not even throw away the hair on her hairbrush for fear of losing something important. She realised that this fear was a problem and was not in reality a risk but still felt the overwhelming urge to check everything and felt concerned when she disposed of any item.

After hearing about someone with similar problems through her network of friends, Anusha sought help from a self-help group run by an OCD charity. Here she learned about ERP and started to implement this herself with the support of the group. She also learned that only certain antidepressants are helpful for OCD symptoms and not all of them. The medications which are useful for both OCD and depression are those known as serotonin reuptake inhibitors.

Once again, Anusha's story demonstrates how OCD compulsive behaviour can mimic Hoarding Disorder but that the main issue with this is that the person does not have an overwhelming attachment to the items themselves but hoards items directly due to their obsessive fears.

Some people do have both OCD and a true Hoarding Disorder, and this distinction is important to make as in these situations it is important that treatment addresses both problems. The treatment ERP is effective in

OCD, as are the serotonin reuptake inhibiting medications mentioned in Chapter 7. In the past, it has often been said that people with OCD and hoarding do not respond as well to treatment. This is because of the confusion regarding the different approaches to OCD and Hoarding Disorder. It is therefore unsurprising that people with Hoarding Disorder may not respond well to treatment which is designed for OCD and not their hoarding issues. Hoarding Disorder co-existing with OCD is demonstrated by the story of Ahmed.

Ahmed's Story

Ahmed is a 70-year-old man who worked all his life as a warehouse security guard and night watchman until he retired aged 65 years. He had lived alone in a one-bedroomed council flat for several decades and had never married or had children. Over the years, he had been treated for OCD. His OCD concerned having horrible thoughts and images of himself being violent to other people. Ahmed was a gentle and peaceful man, and these thoughts were deeply upsetting to him. He had received three successful bouts of ERP treatment for his OCD but had deteriorated after several years on each occasion when he had fallen ill with his asthma. Whilst being treated for his OCD, he learned that, because these violent thoughts were so opposed to his moral standards and because he found them so distressing, he was not in reality a risk to others but in fact was the opposite and the least likely person to be aggressive. He thus learned to distinguish his thoughts as obsessive thoughts rather than a real threat to anyone.

Over the past 3 years, however, some of his neighbours started complaining that there were several boxes piling up in the communal areas outside Ahmed's flat. At first, the neighbours spoke to Ahmed about this. He was apologetic and promised he would move the items soon. Despite the passing of several months and also several neighbours discussing how these boxes were a trip hazard, nothing happened. Eventually, the council was contacted, and an inspector told Ahmed he needed to move these items as they could be dangerous in the case of fire. Again, nothing happened, so the council issued notice to Ahmed that these items would be removed by them and destroyed.

This caused Ahmed extreme alarm. He decided to contact the therapist who had helped him in the past with his OCD. His therapist contacted his doctor and asked her to make a referral back to their service so that he could assess the situation fully. He then asked Ahmed to contact the council and agree they could liaise with his therapist. Initially, Ahmed was very reluctant to do this but then realised that this would be the only way to control the situation. The therapist arranged to make a home visit. Ahmed was extremely reluctant but, when he was told that otherwise the council might insist and could clear items if they considered them a risk, he reluctantly agreed.

When the therapist visited the home, he was shocked at the state of Ahmed's flat. His heating was not accessible due to the accumulation of newspapers, books, clothes, and other items Ahmed had bought, mainly from charity shops, and which he was insistent were important and might be useful. He had been unable to sleep in his bed or sit on his sofa for many years due to them being piled up with possessions. His bath was also full, and it was clear that Ahmed was only keeping himself clean by washing in the kitchen sink. Despite how hoarded the area was, Ahmed had kept the area around the cooker clear of items, so there was no immediate threat of fire.

The cold damp flat without heating, and covered in dust as effective cleaning was impossible, had worsened Ahmed's asthma and had been a contributing factor to his physical ill health relapses and the subsequent relapse of his OCD symptoms.

The therapist explained to Ahmed how treatment for Hoarding Disorder differed from the ERP for OCD but did have some similarities in that Ahmed would need to face his fear of disposing of objects in order to overcome the problem and live in a comfortable, clean, and healthy flat. Although he dreaded the thought of giving away some of his possessions, Ahmed could see it was necessary if he was to avoid possible eviction by the council.

Clearing his flat in a structured way (as discussed in Chapter 10) took almost a year. After the first few sessions with the therapist, Ahmed was able to proceed on his own but he still had regular meetings with his therapist to discuss his progress and to revisit the advantages of undertaking this clearance himself rather than others forcibly disposing of items.

The real-life stories above demonstrate how hoarding may be a symptom of OCD as a reaction to obsessive thoughts or, as in the story of Ahmed, may be a completely separate diagnosis. Sometimes it is not immediately obvious which of these is the case for an individual. If in doubt, it is usually best to start by tackling the OCD fears and then see what problems remain.

Obsessive Compulsive Personality Disorder

OCPD is a very common type of personality disorder which has been estimated to occur in between 1.9 per cent and 7.8 per cent of the population.[2] It is described in DSM-5-TR as being an enduring personality type which is characterised by the following traits and results in significant distress of interference in day-to-day functioning.

- **Preoccupation with details**

This means that the person struggles with details which are not really important to the overall task or picture.

- **Perfectionism which interferes with a person's ability to complete a task**

Where it is important that the things we do are "good enough", if an individual tries to always be perfect, then they are doomed to failure at least some of the time. Striving for perfection takes time and prevents other things of equal or greater importance from being achieved.

- **Rigidity and unwillingness to change or adapt their opinion**

Whereas most people have some strongly held views on morals, religion, politics, and other issues, in our interaction with others at work, in the family, or socially, not all opinions can be rigidly held at all times. Compromise is often important, and this may be extremely difficult or impossible for someone with OCPD.

- **Reluctance to delegate**

Someone with OCPD may do everything themselves as they feel that other people do not achieve the very high standards that they desire.

- **Excessive conscientiousness and excessive concern about minor details and rules**

Rather than looking at the broader picture, a person with OCPD may get caught up on minor issues which can impair the completion of a task.

- **"Workaholic"**

From time to time, many of us need to work hard and go beyond what would normally be expected in the workplace. Someone with OCPD may always be working extremely hard and staying later than his/her colleagues in the workplace.

- **Reluctance to spend money even on necessities**

People with OCPD may be very reluctant to spend money even on things that are essential for a comfortable and healthy life.

- **Hoarding**

Hoarding is very frequent in OCPD. The hoarding normally involves a reluctance to throw away or discard items that are no longer fully serviceable.

People with OCPD are often distressed by the condition. Sometimes people with OCD can appear to have OCPD due to their symptoms of perfectionism or rigidity, but whereas in OCD symptoms may vary from time to time in severity, in OCPD the symptoms tend to be more consistent and deeply "ingrained" in the character.

It is also clear that OCPD may be confused with Hoarding Disorder. Not only do people with OCPD often hoard items but also symptoms such as being a workaholic and perfectionism can lead to the social isolation that is associated with Hoarding Disorder. The characteristics of both disorders are shown in Table 5.1.

Table 5.1 Hoarding Disorder and OCPD

Hoarding Disorder	OCPD
Persistent feeling of the need to save items irrespective of their monetary value	Need to save items in order to save money
Unable to discard possessions due to strong emotional bond with items	Not such strong emotional bond to items
Cluttered living space	Living space may be cluttered due to hoarded items
Depression	Depression is common
Loneliness and social isolation	People with OCPD are often socially isolated and lonely

As can be seen, the symptoms of both disorders do overlap to a great extent, but it is the additional symptoms of OCPD with perfectionism, pedantry, excessively hard-working, and intolerance of imperfections in others which help distinguish the conditions.

The story of Ciaran demonstrates OCPD and how it has impacted on his life.

Ciaran's Story

Ciaran is a 45-year-old man who has a PhD qualification in astrophysics and lives with his parents in a three-bedroomed semi-detached house in the suburbs. His parents are in their 80s and are both retired but they have to cook for Ciaran as well as help him with his self-care activities such as washing and dressing. In addition, Ciaran refuses to throw away any books or exercise pads, and has every scrap of paper he has used since his first time at school aged 4. Consequently, his bedroom was extremely overcrowded, and he was unable to sleep on the bed as it was covered in boxes of books and papers. As a result, his parents recently purchased a large shed for the garden where Ciaran keeps some of his papers in boxes as well as having boxes in all other rooms of the house.

As the only child, Ciaran was always the pride of both his parents. He was an extremely clever and bright child who was meticulous in his work and would spend hours and hours correcting his work. At school, his insistence on his work being totally correct did not impair him too much, although the require-ment meant he had little time for playing and socialising and had few friends. After school he went on to university, where again he spent most of his time working and ensuring his work was perfect and that he gained good exami-nation results. He did not enjoy not gaining 100 per cent in every examination, but was relatively content provided he was top of the class.

After he left university, Ciaran went to work for a large engineering firm who had head-hunted him for his outstanding intellectual and academic per-formance. It was here in the workplace that things started to really go wrong for him. He had various people who were working with him, but Ciaran was extremely difficult to work with. He constantly berated his junior colleagues about the poor standard of their work. He would start work at 6:00am and often would not leave until after 8:00pm. He criticised others in the workplace for their "lack of commitment". Constantly doing all the work himself, Ciaran was unable to delegate. In addition, if someone had a different idea about how a project might run, Ciaran would become angry and sarcastic and would refuse to speak to the person who had made the new suggestion. After 5 years, Ciaran lost his job following multiple complaints and several official warnings about his behaviour.

Having lost his job, Ciaran returned to his parent's house. He spent much of his time in the first few years trying to sue the company for "unfair dismissal" but was unsuccessful after multiple attempts. Without his work, Ciaran appeared to become increasingly miserable and so embarked on his PhD and worked on this on-line as he felt unable to face a workplace environment again. This took him 12 years due to his meticulous attention to detail. Gaining his PhD at the age of 40, Ciaran was again left without a job or study. He had always been fussy about his personal hygiene but began to spend increasing time in the bathroom to ensure he was perfectly clean. He had no obsessive thoughts about contamination or other fears, but just felt that he wished to be "perfectly clean". As this progressed, he reached the stage when he felt unable to do this on his own, and asked his mother or father to accompany him to the bathroom, where he would have a lengthy bath followed by a shower three times a day. His parents were asked to observe these procedures, which could take up to an hour each time. Ciaran became very irritated with them as he felt they did not always give this their full attention, and this resulted in multiple loud family arguments.

His mother attended her GP recently to have a routine check-up. and it was noticed that she was looking stressed and unwell. When asked about this, she broke down and explained all the chores she was having to do at home for Ciaran. It was suggested that Ciaran should seek help for his condition, but his mother was frightened he would become angry. Eventually, it was agreed that the GP would ask Ciaran to make an appointment to see the GP for a check-up. Ciaran did see the GP and very reluctantly agreed to be seen by the local mental health services as he felt this would "prove there's nothing wrong with me". Ciaran is currently seeing a therapist for help with his OCPD.

Treatment of OCPD is not well researched. There is evidence that treatment with the same type of medication used for OCD, the serotonin reuptake inhibitors, can be helpful in the high doses that are also used in OCD. A talking therapy called Psychodynamic Psychotherapy has been reported to be useful for some people. There is more evidence for Cognitive Behaviour Therapy (CBT), where the therapist and patient work together to discover current themes in the individual's thinking which may be unhelpful, and to work out if they can find more productive ways of thinking which will help them to achieve their aims in life.

The story of Ciaran demonstrates some of the differences between pure Hoarding Disorder, hoarding complicating OCD, and hoarding as an integral part of OCPD.

KEY POINTS

- A high proportion of people with Hoarding Disorder also have OCD.

- People with OCD as well as having Hoarding Disorder may hoard items due to their obsessive thoughts and worries.

- Obsessive Compulsive Personality Disorder (OCPD) can often be mistaken for OCD. The key difference is that, unlike in OCD, the perfectionistic and controlling behaviours are deeply ingrained and seem to be part of the individual's character.

- In OCD, the symptoms are more likely to wax and wane than in OCPD.

- Hoarding is one of the main symptoms of OCPD.

- The hoarding in OCPD is often related to a resistance to spend money or may be related to perfectionism, which is very common in OCPD.

- The treatment of people with OCD and OCPD with hoarding symptoms is different from treatment of Hoarding Disorder.

6

· · · · · · ·

Hoarding in People with Attention Deficit Hyperactivity Disorder, Autism, and Impulse Control Issues

In this chapter, we will examine the substantial overlap, similarities, and also connections between people with Hoarding Disorder, Obsessive Compulsive Personality Disorder (OCPD), Attention Deficit Hyperactivity Disorder (ADHD), and Autistic Spectrum Disorder (ASD). The importance of ADHD in many people with hoarding will be examined along with a discussion about how the increasing recognition of a link between the two conditions has led to research into new ways of treating Hoarding Disorder. It is also recognised that autism interacts with hoarding as well as ADHD in a number of ways. Some people with autism are unable to tolerate any clutter at all whilst others hoard huge numbers of items due to difficulty in decision making. In addition, a substantial proportion of people with autism also have a diagnosis of Obsessive Compulsive Disorder (OCD). As has already been discussed (Chapter 5), OCD may present with hoarding symptoms due to the nature of obsessive thoughts as well as Hoarding Disorder.

Although Hoarding Disorder has often been included and associated with OCD, it is now increasingly apparent that many people with Hoarding Disorder often have an inability to fully concentrate on issues, and many other features of ADHD. Indeed, there is considerable overlap in the diagnoses of Hoarding Disorder, OCPD, ADHD, and Autistic Spectrum Disorder (ASD).

Examples of the overlaps are shown in Table 6.1.

Table 6.1 Similarities and overlap between Hoarding Disorder, OCPD, ADHD, and ASD

Symptom	Hoarding Disorder	OCPD	ADHD	ASD
Social and communication issues which may lead to social isolation	Frequent	Frequent	Very frequent due to hyperactivity	Very frequent
Sensitivity to intensity of or specific tastes, smells, sounds, textures	Not usually	Not usually	Can occur as people with ADHD are often attracted to specific sensations for stimulation	Very frequent
Liking sameness and routine	Sometimes	Frequent	People with ADHD may be attracted to familiarity and sameness as a way of controlling their heightened emotions	Very frequent
Fixated on a specific issue or hobby	Sometimes	Frequent	People with ADHD may get periods of excessive focussing on a particular issue or subject	Very frequent
Perfectionism	Very frequent	Very frequent	Sometimes	Sometimes

Symptom	Hoarding Disorder	OCPD	ADHD	ASD
Workaholic	Sometimes	Very frequent	May occur as a function of intense interest in one area of life	May occur as a function of intense interest in one area of life
Lack of flexibility	Very frequent	Very frequent	May occur as a function of being unable to attend to others	Very frequent
Miserliness	Very frequent	Very frequent	Not usually	May occur due to lack of social awareness
Inability to delegate jobs to others	Not usually	Very frequent	Not usually	May occur due to lack of social awareness
Inability to demonstrate affection	Not usually	Very frequent	Whereas people with ADHD experience affection, their inability to concentrate may mean that it is not demonstrated	Very frequent
Preoccupation with details	Very frequent	Very frequent	May occur as a function of "hyperfocus" on a specific topic	Very frequent
Difficulty in sorting and classifying objects	Very frequent	Very frequent	Frequent due to lack of concentration and attention	Very frequent
Difficulty and extreme distress in discarding items	Very frequent	Very frequent	Very frequent	Very frequent and can be related to liking sameness

Table 6.1 (Cont.)

Symptom	Hoarding Disorder	OCPD	ADHD	ASD
Living in a cluttered environment	Very frequent	Very frequent	Very frequent	Frequent if environment not controlled by others
Social isolation	Very frequent	Very frequent	Very frequent	Very frequent
Loneliness	Very frequent	Very frequent	Very frequent	Very frequent
Anxiety	Very frequent	Very frequent	Very frequent	Very frequent
Depression	Very frequent	Very frequent	Very frequent	Very frequent
Lack of attention and concentration	Not usually	Not usually	Always	Not usually
Hyperactivity	Not usually	Not usually	Always	Frequently the self-soothing activities may appear to be hyperactivity

Table 6.1 demonstrates that any of the symptoms associated with Hoarding Disorder, OCPD, ADHD, and ASD can occur in any of the four conditions.

Attention Deficit Hyperactivity Disorder

Attention Deficit Hyperactivity Disorder (ADHD) can be diagnosed in both children and adults. It starts in childhood but may be overlooked, and children with ADHD have often been labelled as disruptive and naughty in the past and may, as a result, have failed to achieve their potential in school and beyond.

The main symptoms of ADHD as described in the *Diagnostic and Statistical Manual of Mental Disorders*, 5th Edition, Text Revision (DSM-5-TR) fall into two main categories:

- **Lack of attention (at least six of the following for children and five for adults for a diagnosis)**
  - Not paying attention and making careless mistakes in school, work, etc.
  - Difficulty in maintaining concentration on work or play.
  - Appears not to listen when being spoken to.
  - Often starts a piece of work but fails to complete it or has difficulty following through instructions.
  - Difficulty in organising things.
  - Avoids or dislikes tasks that need deep concentration.
  - Often loses things that are needed for the task in hand.
  - Easily distracted by other things going on.
  - Forgetful in daily activities.

- **Hyperactivity/impulsivity (at least six of the following for children and five for adults for a diagnosis)**
  - Fidgeting or tapping movements of feet and arms.
  - Often gets up from seat when expected to sit still.
  - Runs around or is active in situations where this is not appropriate.
  - Noisy in activities where may be expected to be quiet.
  - Seems to be always moving.
  - Talks excessively.
  - Blurts out answers before the other person has finished their question.
  - Difficulty in waiting for their turn.
  - Interrupts and intrudes on others inappropriately.

In addition, to make a diagnosis, these symptoms need to have been present since before the age of 12 years and to be present in more than one setting (e.g., school and home). They also need to impair the person's ability at school, work, etc.

Just looking at the description of ADHD it is clear how hoarding may arise as well as a separate diagnosis of Hoarding Disorder occurring. Studies of people with ADHD have found that up to a fifth of them have significant problems with hoarding, and most people with ADHD have more problems than the general population.

The main features of ADHD which result in hoarding are:

- **Difficulties in decision making and organisation**

Many people with ADHD have problems with making decisions in addition to their difficulty in focussing.

- **Impulsivity**

People with ADHD are often impulsive, and this may lead to excessive and unnecessary purchasing of items.

- **Difficulties in concentration and distractibility**

Due to the individual's distractibility and difficulty in focussing on a task, many people with ADHD have problems in sorting their possessions and discarding them.

- **Emotional attachment**

People with ADHD may become overly attached to certain objects and be unable to discard them. This can be due to the fact that people with ADHD may seek out strong sensations and become emotionally attached to objects which provide them with these sensations. Also, the way some people with ADHD become overly focussed on specific things or interests may lead to high emotional attachment to some objects in addition to difficulties in categorisation and decision making that impair the discarding of objects. Finally, some people with ADHD struggle with their emotions and may therefore become emotionally attached to specific objects and possessions.

The story of Claude demonstrates some of these issues.

Claude is a 25-year-old man who lives with his parents in a large house in the country. His father is a highly successful businessman, and his mother works in his father's company. Claude was sent to private schools from the age of 4, but very quickly he was recognised as having behavioural problems. Thereafter, he was asked to leave several schools due to his disruptive behaviour. Unsurprisingly, he did poorly academically.

Eventually his father arranged for Claude to have a personal tutor, but this was equally unsuccessful. Claude became miserable being away from social contacts and still could not learn as he was asked. The tutor suggested that Claude should be assessed by an educational psychologist, but his father was adamant this was unnecessary. His father said that he himself had experienced problems at school and had only learnt to read fluently after leaving school.

Claude stopped education at age 16 with no qualifications. He started working for his father's company, but this was unsuccessful. Claude was always late, never paid attention, and was generally only tolerated because he was the boss's son. After 3 years of trying to get his son settled, his father asked Claude what he wanted to do. Having no clear plan, Claude suggested that he should be given a small allowance and that he would travel around the world. Short of any better ideas apart from disowning his son, which his father did not want to do, there appeared no other options. For the next 5 years, Claude travelled around the world living rough and back-packing. He experimented with various illegal drugs and ended up being arrested for possession of illegal substances and incarcerated in prison. His father paid for the best lawyers, and he was released on a technicality of the law.

Back at home, his parents were despairing as, at 24 years old, he had no education and no job. Claude spent much of his time at home playing computer games and occasionally going out for the night with friends. It was at this time that his mother started talking to him about the huge amount of clutter Claude had in his room. In the past, his room had been untidy and cluttered, but his parents had assumed it was because he was "a messy teenager". They felt he should have improved now he was an adult. His room was packed with clothes so that it was difficult for him to sleep on the bed. Any money he received from his parents he spent on clothes, many of which he didn't wear. After several family rows, his father decided to stop his allowance. A few weeks after this, Claude was arrested for stealing a shirt from the village shop. This time his father decided that he would let Claude face the consequences of his actions. He appeared in court but, as it was a first offence, was given a Community Service order and was to work in the area cleaning up litter. Surprisingly, Claude enjoyed this and got on well with the probation officer assigned to him. This probation officer arranged for Claude to have an assessment at the neurodiversity clinic run by the mental health services of the nearest city.

Claude was diagnosed with ADHD and was offered treatment with the stimulant drug methylphenidate (Ritalin), which greatly improved his thinking and ability to concentrate. He worked with a therapist who helped him with his relationship with his family, and his mother helped him to clear his room.

Having discovered his passion for keeping the natural environment clean and tidy, Claude is now apprenticed to a local garden firm and doing well with his job of cutting grass and pruning. He hopes to one day set up his own business like his father.

The story of Claude demonstrates how ADHD can often go for years undiagnosed and can, in extreme cases, lead to criminal behaviour. Indeed, it has been shown in many Western countries that up to 40 per cent of prisoners meet criteria for ADHD. Of course, only a tiny fraction of people with ADHD break the law, but other issues such as higher risk of accidents due to lack of attention make it really important that this diagnosis is made early.

Autistic Spectrum Disorder and Hoarding

Studies of children and young people who have ASD have reported that up to almost a third have problems with excessive accumulation and hoarding.

ASD has many presentations but key areas for the diagnosis include:

- Social and communication issues.
- Either very high or sometimes low sensitivity to the situation, for example, cannot tolerate loud noise or certain textures and tastes, etc.
- Liking things to not change and to stay consistent and constant, for example, in their home environment or in their personal routines.
- Becoming very fixated in specific interests such as a particular hobby or a particular subject. People with autism can become extreme experts on the things that interest them.

With respect to hoarding, for some individuals with ASD, the idea of clutter and mess or things not being tidy and symmetrical is very difficult, so these are people who are extremely unlikely to hoard. For others, there are four main reasons why they may hoard:

Firstly, people with autism may also have a separate diagnosis of Hoarding Disorder. Similarly, a proportion of people with ASD also have a diagnosis of OCD. As we have seen in the previous chapter, OCD and hoarding can often be found together.

Secondly, the extreme interest in a particular subject or issue may result in hoarding in some individuals.

Thirdly, people with autism sometimes have difficulties in making decisions. This can be due to trying to make a perfect decision and is similar to the perfectionism discussed in the section on OCPD. In addition, they may have difficulty in categorising and sorting their possessions and then in discarding them. It will be seen that this may result in excessive hoarding. The overlaps between these difficulties and Hoarding Disorder are not clear-cut and indeed may not matter as treatment is likely to be similar.

Finally, the social isolation experienced by many people with ASD due to their difficulties in social situations, and a difficulty in grasping meaning from other people's verbal or non-verbal behaviour, results in a situation where it is easy for the individual to hoard items as they may often live alone and without others to help them control the tendency. Also, if in addition the individual has extreme interests or difficulty in categorising items, then it is obvious that a problematic hoard may be developed.

From the above description, it can be seen that there are huge overlaps between hoarding in ADHD, ASD, OCPD, which is often confused with ASD and vice versa, and Hoarding Disorder. Rather than getting caught up in these difficulties in making a clear distinction, it is better to discuss with the individual how they view their hoarding problem and what help they need. The overlap between these three conditions is shown in Table 6.1.

It is important to understand that Table 6.1 only shows some of the picture. Not everyone has all of these symptoms and people are different in their symptoms, the severity of symptoms, and how they present their problems and difficulties.

One of the major findings in children, young people, and adults with ASD is that those with hoarding symptoms also seem to have the worst anxiety and depressive symptoms.

The story of Gina illustrates some of the problems presenting in a young woman with ASD who was not thought to have Hoarding Disorder but who did have significant hoarding problems.

Gina's Story

Gina is a 25-year-old woman who lives in a hostel for people with ASD. Despite being diagnosed with a mild learning disability as well as her autism, she has made huge improvements since living in the hostel and has managed to work for a few hours a week in the communal kitchen where she helps with the preparation of salads that are given to the residents.

Passionate about football (soccer), she collected football programmes and souvenirs from any time she managed to go and see her favourite women's team play. This meant that she had accumulated many items as she also collected anything that reminded her of the day such as tickets for the game, train tickets to get to the match, and even empty drinks cans and food wrappers that she had bought in the stadium.

The staff became concerned about the crowding of items in her room and also felt that keeping food wrappers was unhygienic. However, when they told Gina that she needed to throw some of these items away, she became extremely upset and had a meltdown.

Gina was very fond of all of these items as they reminded her of the happy times she had had at matches, and the thought of losing any of these was extremely distressing to her. One of the staff members, Maggie, was also a football fan and had accompanied Gina to matches. Maggie understood Gina's attachment to these items and was sympathetic to her plight. Maggie thought about this issue and suggested to Gina that they create some scrapbooks for each of the matches she had been to and also separate scrapbooks containing information on each of her favourite players. Gina was keen on this idea, and Maggie took her into town where they could buy some suitable scrapbooks. The pair were then able to sort through the hoard of items. Gina soon discovered that she couldn't remember which match she had bought certain drink cans or food wrappers from. Initially, she was still reluctant to part with these items, but, at Maggie's suggestion, she put them in a plastic bag to think about later.

As the weeks progressed, Gina's room became much tidier. She had several scrapbooks of her mementoes as well as pictures of her favourite players on the walls. Now delighted with her room, Gina would even invite other residents and staff to visit to take a look. Maggie then discussed with Gina how she might go further and get rid of the plastic bags containing empty cans and food wrappers, and this time Gina reluctantly agreed; she realised it did spoil the room she was now so proud of.

This story shows how Gina had a significant problem with hoarding but did not suffer from Hoarding Disorder. The story of Elspeth, who was diagnosed with both ASD and Hoarding Disorder, shows a somewhat different picture.

Elspeth's Story

Elspeth is a 55-year-old woman who lives alone in a two-bedroomed house on the coast. She worked as an office and general cleaner and was known to be very efficient at her job and had excellent references from all her employers.

Unfortunately, Elspeth was diagnosed with breast cancer during a routine mammography and was required to have surgery. Her sister, Maud, whom Elspeth would visit but who on Elspeth's insistence wouldn't visit her, agreed to come and care for her post-operatively. Elspeth was distressed at the idea of her sister coming to stay and suggested that she might like to stay in a local hotel instead and visit her in hospital. Maud was her older sister and had always had a more dominant personality and was insistent that she would stay and help Elspeth in the house as she recuperated. Elspeth eventually agreed Maud could stay but kept on repeating to Maud that she must not touch any of her belongings. Maud was confused by this request and agreed she would not touch anything without Elspeth's permission.

When Maud arrived the day before Elspeth's operation was scheduled, she went to the house. It was a sunny, warm day and Elspeth kept on suggesting that she might like to sit outside. Maud explained she was tired after her journey and wished to have a shower and change her clothes. When she entered the house, Maud could not believe what she saw. The entire house was cluttered with a variety of items; papers and other items covered much of the floor space up to waist height with narrow "corridors" between the piles of objects. There was one place to sit on the sofa in the living room as all other areas were covered with items. One of the bedrooms was totally covered with items so that the bed was not accessible, and the other had a narrow pathway to the bed which was clear of items. The bathroom and kitchen were relatively clear with just a few items on the workspace. When Maud asked Elspeth what all these items were, she explained that her employers would throw away many items such as books, magazines, old coffee cups, and office equipment. Elspeth said that these items might be useful or important. Instead of clearing the rubbish and taking it down to the large rubbish containers in the car park, she took them all home as she was going to "sort them all out". Although Elspeth said she was going to sort the items and dispose of those that were not useful, it was clear that this had never occurred.

Maud suggested that they should both stay in a hotel whilst Elspeth recuperated and that she would order a skip to dispose of all the items. Elspeth became extremely upset at this suggestion. Apart from visiting her sister, she had never stayed anywhere other than her own house since she moved in when she left their parents' home 30 years earlier. She had only agreed to have surgery on the basis that she would be allowed home that evening. Fortunately, the surgeon agreed as she did not require an extensive operation. If he had not agreed, she would have refused surgery despite the consequences of this. This insistence of sameness and the need to be in a familiar environment had been present since early childhood, as had an insistence on a routine. Her attachment to her hoarded items was a shock to Maud, but she recognised that Elspeth had always had difficulty as a child at home when her parents would throw away items. Elspeth now was distraught and was insistent that all of the items were precious and valuable and that she could not part with any of them. Being unsure what to do about this, Maud agreed to stay on her own in a hotel for a few nights and allow Elspeth to sleep in her bed.

The following day when Elspeth went into the hospital for her surgery, Maud asked to speak to a member of the surgical team. She explained the situation to them. The surgical team said that it was not safe for Elspeth to be discharged without an adult who would stay with her overnight following surgery in case of complications. Maud then said she would stay with Elspeth and would sit up on the sofa whilst Elspeth slept in her bed.

The surgery went well, and Elspeth was discharged home. Maud sat with her all night and then left her to go to the hotel and have a rest during the day.

Maud spoke with Elspeth's general practitioner (GP) and discovered that Elspeth was unknown to mental health services. A diagnosis of autism had been made 20 years ago, but since then Elspeth had been discharged from services. The GP said he would contact mental health services and ask for an assessment appointment at home.

Elspeth was not happy about being seen by mental health services but reluctantly agreed when Maud insisted. Maud stayed overnight in the hotel and visited her sister during the day for a week before she returned home. She agreed to visit again at the time of the mental health assessment.

A few weeks later, Elspeth received an appointment from mental health services. The first visit was at the services community base, and Maud attended with Elspeth. Although Elspeth was insistent there was no problem, Maud gave a description and showed photographs of the cluttered home. They were told that a treatment group based on CBT principles would soon be starting and that this would offer a good start to Elspeth's treatment. The idea of being in a group like this was very frightening for Elspeth, who had social anxiety and avoided all social situations. A therapist then agreed to see her for therapy but explained this was likely to mean a longer wait. Ideally, the therapist explained, it would be better if Elspeth had someone that would help her with clearing her house during treatment as any therapist would be unlikely to be able to be there sufficiently often to help Elspeth deal with her hoard. Although some people do manage to do this alone, it was explained it would be easier if someone else was involved. Maud suggested that Elspeth could buy a tablet so that Maud could communicate via videocalls to Elspeth and check on her progress. In this way, she could also join in on the therapy sessions when required. Elspeth accepted this, as she felt her sister was the only person that understood her.

As you can see, it is difficult to distinguish between those who hoard due to their autistic symptoms of having extreme interests and like of familiarity and sameness, and those who have ASD and also a separate Hoarding Disorder. The question of whether this distinction matters or not is also not always clear. In terms of medication, this would be unlikely to help someone with autism and hoarding symptoms, whereas it may be helpful in people with a diagnosis of Hoarding Disorder. Psychological treatment in all cases involves working with the individual in their setting to resolve any issues. Frequently, people with hoarding do not see it as a problem; the role of therapy is trying to walk on the tightrope between keeping the person safe in their environment and not being at risk of eviction, fire, falls, crush injuries, or other harm, and the individual's wishes. A pragmatic approach as shown at the end of this book in Chapter 11 is probably the best way forward. This should be guided as much as possible by the wishes of the person with autism, and may involve some compromises.

KEY POINTS

- There is a huge overlap in the symptoms found in Hoarding Disorder, OCPD, ADHD, and ASD. Almost all of the major symptoms of any of these conditions can be found in the others.

- Anxiety and depression are almost universal at some time in people with ADHD and ASD, and these symptoms seem to drive and worsen hoarding symptoms.

- In addition to overlap in symptoms, Hoarding Disorder itself can also occur in people with ADHD and ASD.

- People with ADHD may hoard items due to excessive emotional attachment to items, as their behaviour can lead them to be isolated from others and form strong attachments to inanimate objects.

- Also, people with ADHD may hoard items due to an inability to classify and sort their possessions.

- The most common problem with hoarding in ADHD is difficulty in concentrating sufficiently to dispose of unnecessary items.

- People with ASD may either excessively hoard or intensely dislike a hoarded environment.

- People with ASD may have symptoms of hoarding, due to a high proportion of people with ASD also having OCD symptoms.

- Main reasons why people with ASD but without a separate diagnosis of Hoarding Disorder or OCD may hoard items include an intense interest in a subject, inability to classify and sort items, over-attachment to inanimate objects due to social interaction difficulties, and liking sameness and an unchanged environment.

7
• • • • • • •

Treatment of Hoarding Disorder: Medication

In this chapter, we will examine the evidence for the various treatments for Hoarding Disorder using medication. The action of the various chemicals in the brain as well as why it is thought they may be useful in Hoarding Disorder is then explored. Full lists of optimal dosages as well as side effects are given. Finally, the possibility of other medications, which are largely unexplored, but which may be useful in the future, is examined.

It has already been noted that, prior to 2013, people with Hoarding Disorder were generally diagnosed as having either Obsessive Compulsive Personality Disorder (OCPD) or Obsessive Compulsive Disorder (OCD). This means that many earlier studies of Hoarding Disorder include people with these diagnoses. When treatments which are known to be useful for OCD were studied in people with hoarding or Hoarding Disorder, it is difficult to determine whether improvements were due to improvements in the OCD symptoms or the Hoarding Disorder itself. It was often noted that people with OCD and hoarding tended to not do as well with treatment as those without hoarding. This finding is unsurprising when you consider that the treatments being used were geared to improve OCD and not specifically directed towards the hoarding symptoms themselves! Now that Hoarding Disorder is recognised as a diagnosis in its own right, there are more studies which are examining Hoarding Disorder itself without OCD or other conditions. This will mean that, in the future, more targeted treatments will be available for Hoarding Disorder. At present, there are some tried and tested treatments which are known to be helpful, and these will form the basis of this chapter. It is important to note that, at present, there are far more studies examining the effect of psychological treatment rather than medication.

Medication and Hoarding Disorder

Most medications which are found to be useful for various psychological symptoms act via chemicals known as neurotransmitters. These are chemicals which act as messengers and allow the brain to transmit information from one cell to another. These neurotransmitter circuits are extremely complex and some of the medications may act on more than one of the systems. Simply put, the four systems we will look at are the *serotonin system* which tends to operate mainly at the front, or what is known as the forebrain; the *dopamine system* which operates mainly in the lower part of the forebrain and midbrain; the *norepinephrine system* which also operates mainly in the forebrain as well as midbrain; and lastly the *glutamate system*, which is distributed widely throughout the brain and which has a somewhat different action of modulating or controlling the actions of other neurotransmitters. In the simplest of terms, the forebrain is what is involved in emotions and the fight or flight reaction, amongst many other functions. The midbrain has an important function in relaying information between the forebrain and hindbrain and also as part of the reward system in the brain (which lies in the forebrain and midbrain). The hindbrain is involved in functions which keep us alive, such as breathing and sleeping.

Medication is rarely the first-line treatment in Hoarding Disorder, but there is evidence that certain medications may help in a problem which is often very difficult for the person to recognise in themselves and to come forward for treatment. This reluctance to come forward for treatment is undoubtedly linked to the considerable stigmatisation of the condition in the past when many individuals were made to feel that it was their "fault". This leads to shame and reluctance to admit to a problem. As we study Hoarding Disorder more, we will reduce and eventually smash this stigma.

It is important to note that, whereas these medications may be helpful to individuals, in general there is a lack of research, so it is difficult to fully recommend any particular medicine for Hoarding Disorder. Thus, it must always be a decision made by the individual in consultation with his or her doctor. Additionally, different medications may help with depression, anxiety, obsessive compulsive, or other symptoms which may be present in addition to the hoarding problems.

As with any medication, it is important that these are started in collaboration with a clinician who has fully assessed you. In all cases, if you have been on the medication for any time, do not stop abruptly, as this may result in withdrawal symptoms. It is important to reduce and withdraw the tablets in consultation with your physician.

The various medications which have been used in Hoarding Disorder are shown in Table 7.1. Full descriptions of each of these follows in the text.

Medications Used in OCD Which May Be Helpful for Hoarding Disorder

Clomipramine

Clomipramine may or may not help with Hoarding Disorder. Some studies have suggested it is useful, but these often include people who also have OCD, and it is difficult to tease out the specific effect on hoarding. Clomipramine does have significant side effects as well as other problems, so cannot be recommended as a first-line treatment for Hoarding Disorder. Having said this, some people do find it useful, and if you have

Table 7.1 Medication and Hoarding Disorder

Type of medication	Examples of medication	Brand names	Recommended daily dosage	Comments
Serotonin reuptake inhibitors (SRIs): these consist of clomipramine and also the selective serotonin reuptake inhibitors (SSRIs).	*Clomipramine	Anafranil	225 mg	These drugs are proven beneficial in OCD. Most studies have included people with OCD when used in Hoarding Disorder. Research is mixed but there does appear to be benefit for many.
	**Fluvoxamine	Faverin (UK) Luvox (UK and USA)	Up to 300 mg	Also, useful for the depression that often accompanies Hoarding Disorder.
	Sertraline	Lustral (UK) Zoloft (USA)	Up to 200 mg	*Clomipramine is an older type of drug than the others and has more side effects.
	Fluoxetine	Prozac (UK and USA) Prozep (UK) Olena (UK) Oxactin (UK) Rapiflux (USA) Sarafem (USA) Selfemra (USA)	Up to 60 mg	**Fluvoxamine is the first of the newer serotonin reuptake inhibitors to be developed and may have more side effects than the others (apart from clomipramine) for many people.
	Paroxetine	Seroxat (UK) Paxil (USA) Brisdelle (USA) Pexeva (USA)	40 mg	
	Citalopram	Cipramil (UK and USA)	Up to 40 mg	
	Escitalopram	Cipralex (UK) Lexapro (USA)	Up to 20 mg	

Table 7.1 (Cont.)

Type of medication	Examples of medication	Brand names	Recommended daily dosage	Comments
Dopamine blockers	Risperidone	Risperdal (UK and USA)	0.5 up to 2 mg if helpful	There is currently very little research into whether or not adding a dopamine blocker to SRIs or prescribing dopamine blockers on their own is helpful. Much of the research is based on case history reports rather than properly controlled trials.
	Aripiprazole	Abilify (UK and USA) Maintena (USA) Aristada (USA)	2.5–5 mg	
	Olanzapine	Zyprexa (UK and USA)	2.5–5 mg	
	Quetiapine	Atrolak (UK) Biquelle (UK) Seroquel (UK and USA) Sondate (UK) Zaluron (UK)	25 mg	
Medication with possible specific effects on Hoarding Disorder	Venlafaxine	Efexor (UK and USA) Vensir (UK) Vencarm (UK) Venlafix (UK) Venlablue (UK)	37.5 mg increasing up to 225 mg	This medicine is a serotonin norepinephrine reuptake inhibitor (or SNRI). In general, this has not been shown to be as effective as SRIs in OCD, so the use of SNRIs in small studies of people with Hoarding Disorder with a good outcome is encouraging. In general, SNRIs may have fewer side effects than SRIs.

Table 7.1 (Cont.)

Type of medication	Examples of medication	Brand names	Recommended daily dosage	Comments
	Atomoxetine	Strattera (UK and USA)	40–100 mg	A noradrenaline reuptake inhibitor. Its usage is based on the observation that people with Hoarding Disorder may have problems also with attention, concentration, and/or impulsivity. Only individual case studies in Hoarding Disorder.
	Methylphenidate	Ritalin (UK and USA) Concerta (UK and USA) Delmosart (UK) Equasym (UK) Medikinet (UK) Daytrana (USA) Focalin (USA) Metadate (USA) Quillivant (USA)	10–60 mg in divided dosage with normal dosage 20–30 mg	This is a stimulant widely used for adults with Attention Deficit Hyperactivity Disorder (ADHD). It has been tried in a few individuals with Hoarding Disorder with good effect due to the observation that there may be an overlap between ADHD and Hoarding Disorder.

Table 7.1 (Cont.)

Type of medication	Examples of medication	Brand names	Recommended daily dosage	Comments
Medication which has no proven benefit but which may prove useful with more research	Minocycline	Minocin (UK and USA) Dynacin (USA) Solodyn (USA) Ximino (USA)	50 mg twice daily for 3 days followed by 100 mg twice daily	This is an antibiotic which has been used for many years in the treatment of acne. It acts also on the glutamate system in the brain. Studies on a few individuals with Hoarding Disorder suggest it may help the condition, has few side effects, and was generally well tolerated by individuals who mostly chose to remain on the medication after the study ended.
	Naltrexone	Trexan (UK) Nalerona (UK) Abernil (UK) Naltrexona (UK) Adepend (UK) ReVia (UK and USA) Depade (UK and USA) Vivitrol (UK and USA)		Naltrexone has been used to treat drug and alcohol abuse. It acts by blocking the receptors in the brain that respond to these. It has been tried in the treatment of Hoarding Disorder but there has been little research into its usefulness.

Hoarding Disorder and have received treatment with clomipramine which you have found useful, then you should certainly continue to take it.

In the 1970s, it was discovered that clomipramine had a specific anti-OCD effect. This effect was shown to be independent and unrelated to its anti-depressant effect, although it is also an antidepressant. Clomipramine belongs to a class of drugs known as tricyclic antidepressants, or TCAs. These drugs work on a number of chemicals in the brain. TCAs have been demonstrated to work on the five major chemical systems in the brain which transmit information between brain cells. These chemicals are known as neurotransmitters. Clomipramine has a particularly powerful effect on the serotonin neurotransmitter system (sometimes also known as 5-HT system). It was discovered that clomipramine increased the levels of serotonin in specific areas of the brain. The way clomipramine works is that it blocks the neurotransmitter serotonin from being rapidly taken back into the brain cells, which results in an increase in serotonin. This increase in serotonin seems to be what causes the anti-OCD effect. The parts of the brain that are affected by low levels of serotonin in OCD are in the front of the brain in an area known as the orbito-frontal area.

Although clomipramine is certainly usually effective in reducing some of the symptoms of OCD, it is not without its problems. Because the drug acts on a range of other neurotransmitter systems in the brain, clomipramine has a large number of potential side effects. The more common side effects of clomipramine include:

- Dry mouth
- Dizziness
- Headache
- Constipation
- Difficulty in passing water
- Drowsiness
- Sexual problems
- Weight gain
- Blurred vision

Much less commonly are more serious side effects reported, including the risk of inducing fits. Not everyone has side effects with clomipramine. Introducing the drug at a low dose with gradual increases reduces the risk of experiencing side effects.

Another major disadvantage of clomipramine is that it is extremely dangerous in overdose. For OCD, higher levels of drug are needed than for depression. An effective dose for OCD is usually 225 mg clomipramine a day. Rarely should this be prescribed over 250 mg, although occasionally doses up to 300 mg are used. An accidental or deliberate act of self-poisoning with clomipramine is very dangerous and can be quickly fatal as the drug can have devastating effects on the heart and other organs.

Selective Serotonin Reuptake Inhibiting Drugs

Selective serotonin reuptake inhibitors (SSRIs) are more modern drugs than clomipramine and are effective in treating depression, anxiety, OCD, and many other conditions. In general, they have fewer side effects than the older drugs, such as clomipramine, and are safer in overdosage. Research into their use in Hoarding Disorder has, however, been mixed, with most studies looking at people who have both OCD and hoarding. In some of these studies, it would appear that they have a beneficial effect including on hoarding, but in others, they seem to be less beneficial. Once again, they may be very helpful for people who have Hoarding Disorder, with a beneficial effect on depression, anxiety, and OCD symptoms irre-spective of their effect on hoarding symptoms.

Fluvoxamine was the first SSRI to be generally used and available. Although effective, there are suggestions it may have more side effects than other SSRIs, although it has fewer side effects than clomipramine.

Some of the possible side effects of SSRIs include:

- Feeling energised or agitated or restless, or occasionally drowsiness
- Feeling of nausea

- Not wanting to eat
- Difficulty sleeping
- Diarrhoea
- Dizziness
- Dry mouth
- Sexual problems
- Headache
- Blurred vision

Not everyone experiences side effects with these drugs. Also, starting at a low dose and increasing on a 1–2 weekly basis tends to reduce the risk of experiencing side effects. Although some of the possible side effects of SSRIs are similar to those that can be experienced with clomipramine, the frequencies of these are usually lower. For example, problems with sexual function have been reported in up to 80 per cent of people taking clomipramine but in less than 30 per cent on SSRIs. Another factor is that the common side effects of SSRIs such as feeling nauseous and not wishing to eat usually wear off after 1–2 weeks of starting the medication and do not seem to recur when doses are increased.

Dopamine Blocking Medications

These medicines are often referred to as "antipsychotics" as they are the same medicines which are used to treat people with psychotic disorders such as schizophrenia. In psychoses, however, considerably higher dosages are used than in conditions such as OCD. Indeed, at lower dosages the drugs seem to act in a very different way. These medications act on the dopamine systems rather than primarily the serotonin systems mentioned above. Dopamine acts further towards the midbrain in what is often described as the "reward system" of the brain.

In people with OCD who do not respond to SSRIs, a low dose of a dopamine blocker is usually the next step in treatment. There are older types of dopamine blockers which tend to have many more side effects; in general, the medicines used are known as "atypical" drugs. Several are used in OCD, but the most commonly used are risperidone, aripiprazole, olanzapine, and quetiapine. Side effects with dopamine blockers are much less frequently seen than with the much higher doses used for schizophrenia. There is always a worry about the long-term side effects of a movement disorder. Although only rarely seen in people treated for many years on high-dose antipsychotic medication, developing a movement disorder is very much less likely in the tiny doses used for OCD. Older dopamine blockers are known as conventional antipsychotics, and these tend to have more side effects and sometimes more acute movement disorders can seen but generally at higher doses. People on these drugs should generally have some monitoring of their electrocardiograph (ECG or EKG) because of a very small risk of problems with heart conductivity. Aripiprazole, a newer drug, does not cause any heart conduction changes.

In terms of more common side effects seen, they may include some drowsiness, except for aripiprazole where the opposite can be found. Weight gain can occur, particularly with olanzapine. It must be stressed that these side effects are less problematic due to the low doses used in these conditions.

In OCD, these medications are added to an SSRI and there is no evidence they are useful on their own. The evidence for improvements in people with Hoarding Disorder is also very meagre and based on case reports, so it is another issue when discussing with your doctor and deciding if such treatment may be useful to you or is the best way forward.

Venlafaxine

Venlafaxine is different from the SSRIs and is known as a serotonin norepinephrine reuptake inhibitor (SNRI). Whereas SSRIs mainly act on the serotonin system in the brain which is concentrated in the front of the brain, and dopamine blockers act predominantly on the "reward areas" of the brain, norepinephrine, which is also known as noradrenaline, acts as both a hormone in the body and a neurotransmitter in the brain. As already noted, it operates mainly in the fore (front) brain as well as in part of the midbrain and in particular in what are known as "basal areas".

Venlafaxine is a powerful antidepressant but has also been found to be useful in those people with ADHD. Because ADHD is thought to be associated with Hoarding Disorder in some people, its use in helping people with Hoarding Disorder has been suggested. There have been a few reports of venlafaxine being useful in reducing symptoms of Hoarding Disorder, but these involve small numbers of people and it has not been fully researched.

However, venlafaxine is generally well tolerated, and most people do not experience any side effects. Those who have side effects often report that these improve as their body becomes more used to the medication. Side effects that have been reported include:

- Nausea or feeling sick
- Sweating/hot flushes
- Headaches
- Dry mouth
- Dizzy feelings
- Sleepiness
- Difficulty sleeping
- Constipation

Because venlafaxine has few side effects, it may be worthwhle trying in people who have Hoarding Disorder to see if it can help their symptoms.

Methylphenidate

Methylphenidate is a stimulant drug which is known to be useful for people who have ADHD. As already noted, some people with ADHD seem to also have problems with Hoarding Disorder. Some clinicians have therefore tried this treatment in people with Hoarding Disorder with or without ADHD.

There have only been a few case history studies which suggested that methylphenidate may be helpful in some people with Hoarding Disorder, particularly in helping people reduce their acquisition of new items.

It is really too early to fully support this as a treatment, but again it is something that could be discussed with your physician.

Common side effects of methylphenidate include:

- Headache
- Increased irritability or feeling anxious and tense
- Trouble sleeping
- Loss of appetite
- Stomach ache
- Dry mouth
- Nausea and vomiting

In short, it is difficult to recommend methylphenidate to all people with Hoarding Disorder at this time. It may particularly be helpful to those who have problems with acquiring large numbers of new objects and/or are more impulsive.

Possible Medication in the Future

As has already been stated, there is very little research into medication and Hoarding Disorder, but this is likely to change over the next few years, so it is worthwhile being hopeful for the future.

Examples of medication which may prove useful are listed below:

- **D-Cycloserine**

Theoretically, it has been suggested that this medication may be useful in a range of Obsessive Compulsive and Related Disorders, but there is no research to back this up. D-Cycloserine is an antibiotic originally, but it seems to also have an effect in increasing brain connections and possibly new learning ability. It acts via the glutamate system.

Side effects include over-excitability, dizziness, anxiety, confusion, memory loss, lack of energy, and, extremely rarely, seizures.

- **Minocycline**

This is an antibiotic which has been used long term in the management of acne and other skin conditions. It has been used in conjunction with SSRIs in people with OCD and may have a beneficial effect on hoarding symptoms, but this has not been fully researched. It has the benefit of few side effects and is generally well tolerated. Its main symptoms are related to allergic reactions. Additionally, some people have reported worsening of depression, whereas others have reported improvements in depression.

- **Naltrexone**

This drug is used in the treatment of drug addiction as it acts by blocking the brain's reward system which gives the "buzz" with opioids and similar drugs. Because Hoarding Disorder has sometimes been found to have some similarities with addictions, naltrexone has been tried in a few people. There is no convincing research in this area. Side effects include abdominal or stomach pain and cramps, anxiety, restlessness, trouble sleeping, headache, joint or muscle pains, nausea or vomiting, and unusual tiredness.

In summary, we are in the early days of researching the best medication or combination of medications for Hoarding Disorder, and it is likely we will learn more and have more specific, better tolerated, and more effective treatments in the future.

SUMMARY

- There is little research in the area of Hoarding Disorder and the medications which may be helpful.
- The mainstay of medication treatment is treatment with the antidepressant drugs known as serotonin reuptake inhibitors. These may or may not have a direct effect on hoarding symptoms, but they can help

improve any symptoms of depression, anxiety, or obsessive compulsive symptoms which may complicate the Hoarding Disorder.

- If serotonin reuptake inhibitors do not work, the next stage is usually to add in a dopamine blocker. There is even less work looking at how these impact on Hoarding Disorder, but again they may help the obsessive compulsive and other symptoms if present.

- Venlafaxine is a powerful antidepressant which acts in a different way to the serotonin reuptake inhibitors and may be specifically useful in Hoarding Disorder, but only tiny studies have taken place.

- Some researchers have noted that Hoarding Disorder often overlaps with ADHD and have suggested treatment with stimulants such as methylphenidate may be helpful. Only a few case reports have been performed.

- There are a number of other approaches which are being examined for the treatment of Hoarding Disorder. Some of these are based on a view that Hoarding Disorder is similar to an addiction.

8

• • • • • • •

Treatment of Hoarding Disorder: Psychological Approaches

In this chapter, we will examine the psychological treatments that have been found to be helpful for people with Hoarding Disorder. The main approach used is Cognitive Behaviour Therapy (CBT). This may be with an individual or in a group setting. Although, as with much of the research into Hoarding Disorder, the number of studies of high quality is limited, we have good evidence that CBT does work and can have life-changing impacts both on the hoarding and also on the depressive symptoms which often accompany Hoarding Disorder. One of the major issues, however, can be the reluctance of people with Hoarding Disorder to enter into treatment programmes and then to stick with the programme. There may be many reasons for this reluctance. One recent development which may be hopeful for the future has been using an approach known as Compassion Focussed Therapy (CFT) in addition to the standard CBT.

Cognitive Behaviour Therapy (CBT)

As has already been mentioned, Hoarding Disorder was not recognised as a condition in its own right until the publication of the *Diagnostic and Statistical Manual of Mental Disorders*, 5th Edition (DSM-5) by the American Psychiatric Association in 2013. Prior to this, people with hoarding were classified as having either Obsessive Compulsive Disorder (OCD) or Obsessive Compulsive Personality Disorder, or incorrectly often considered to be making a lifestyle choice. Consequently, there is very little reliable research prior to 2013. Early studies of people with OCD suggested that those with hoarding symptoms may do less well in treatment than those with other symptoms. This is hardly surprising when you consider that Hoarding Disorder was not being separated from OCD (with or without hoarding symptoms); thus, people with pure Hoarding Disorder were not usually receiving specific treatment aimed at the hoarding problems themselves. Since 2013, the situation has changed dramatically, and there are now many studies examining the best way to treat Hoarding Disorder using CBT.

The model of treatment for Hoarding Disorder using CBT focusses on four main areas:

- Avoidance of sorting, making decisions, and discarding items.
- Difficulty in the organisation, categorisation, and decision-making process.
- Emotional attachment to the possessions.
- Hoarding-related beliefs such as concern about catastrophic consequences of making a "wrong" decision and throwing away something you may need.

Some of these issues are targeted at when the sorting and discarding stands to take place, as this is when the worries will be the most prominent.

The main components of CBT treatment for Hoarding Disorder include the following:

- **Psychoeducation about Hoarding Disorder**

This means learning about Hoarding Disorder. It is important that the person starts to understand how their hoarding has developed and how their genes as well as their environment have meant that they have developed the symptoms of the disorder. It is very important that they understand that Hoarding Disorder is not their choice any more than any other condition such as heart disease is a choice but is a condition which they did not choose to have. There is therefore no shame involved in having Hoarding Disorder. Although it is a problematic condition which can be persistent for many decades, there is light at the end of the tunnel, and they can improve and get better. The single most important step anyone with Hoarding Disorder can do is to recognise that they have a problem and to come forward for help. For a person to come forward and to admit to their problem does require a huge amount of inner strength and bravery. Friends and relatives need to understand how very hard this step is to take and the courage it takes to do.

Making sure that the person fully understands their disorder, the possible reasons for its development, and the options for treatment, including understanding that they can get better, is very important in the process of recovery.

- **Working out the cost:benefit analysis of the problem**

Once the person has started to admit to the problem, the next step is to look at the costs and benefits of how they are currently living and of how they would live if they didn't have a hoarding problem. This can be difficult for a person who has lived for many decades in a hoarded environment, as they often cannot remember living in a clutter-free environment. Helpful questions can be "if you had a magic wand and could magic your living space to your ideal, what would it look like?" It is important for them to think of what they would like if they believe they have a "collection". For example, the massive pile of papers filling up every area of the home and where no one can find any specific article: would the relevant interesting articles be cut out and stored in scrapbooks, with irrelevant pages discarded? The piles of clothes covering every item of furniture, muddled up, and not available to wear due to them being crumpled and dishevelled: how would it be to have a selection of neat clothes in a wardrobe or cupboard, and have the money spent on clothes available instead to go out and spend on enjoyable activities wearing smart clothes?

As you can see, the cost:benefit analysis will be different for every person. Someone who has piles of apparently random items because they fear they may need the items in the future may be helped to examine how they may be able to get their hands on similar items in an emergency without storing everything in their home.

Some people will at this point be able to identify the thoughts they have which make it difficult to discard items and make them collect more. By examining these hard, it may be possible to challenge some of the thinking behind the problems. For others, this stage comes later in the course of treatment and only after they start to reduce their hoard.

- **Working collaboratively with the therapist or on your own on a plan of action**

The next task is working out where and how the hoard should be tackled. If there are health and safety issues then those must be addressed as priority, but if the house is cluttered but the cooker and heaters have appropriate space around them and there are no immediate risks, then a choice needs to be made as to which area of the home to concentrate on first. It may be decided, for example, that the person wants to start in their living room, and their goal is for this to be clear and tidy with room for people to sit down on the sofa and to place cups on the coffee table. Another person may want to clear the bath so that they can reward themselves with a long hot soak in the bathtub. After fully assessing risks and tackling any risks first, where to start working is down to the individual's choice. What is important is to choose one area and stick with it. It can be very tempting to flit from room to room and place to place, but in this case, it is much more difficult to see change and the person may become disheartened at their lack of progress and may even give up. Sticking to one area and one room means that progress can be seen more readily.

- **Stopping any further acquisition of items**

Before working on discarding any items, it is vital to stop the collection of any new items. This means placing a *total ban on new items entering the property.* It would be pointless to clear one area of the house, only to find that new items have been obtained to replace the previous hoard. Trying to address hoarding without putting a stop to the acquisition of new items is rather like trying to bail water out of a boat without addressing a large hole in the bottom. This can be a difficult thing for someone with Hoarding Disorder to agree to, but it is an essential step towards treatment and reaching the goals of a functional living space they can be proud of. Of course no one is perfect, and indeed, perfection is not a desirable or possible state for humans, so slip-ups will occur from time to time. It is also important not to catastrophise these slip-ups but to treat them as learning experiences. For example, it may demonstrate that, for example, going to a shopping centre when feeling low and depressed is more likely to lead to a person buying more items. Doing another activity which they find enjoyable, such as walking in the park or visiting a local tea room, may help to lift mood without the risk of buying more things. Purchasing things can have an immediate feeling of reward in the brain, but this can be followed by feelings of guilt and failure. Understanding this can also be important in moving forward in treatment.

- **Learning how to classify, organise, make decisions, and sort items (and dispose of unnecessary items)**

Once the decision has been made on where to start and the ban on new items entering the property has been agreed, it is time to start sorting items. Depending on the nature and content of the hoard, anyone sorting this may need protective clothing. For example, the items are at least likely to be dusty, so dust masks and old clothes may need to be worn. If any items are deteriorating and rotting, then protective gloves and plastic aprons may be needed.

The key to sorting is for the person to select an item and make an immediate decision of whether to keep or discard. This should be an immediate reaction, and it is important the person does not hold on to the item for too long. The longer the person holds on to the item, the more attached to it they are likely to feel. A quick and immediate reaction is usually best. Once a decision has been made to discard, then the item should be placed in a black plastic bag before moving on to the next item. Depending on the contents of the hoard, there may be three potential options of: keep, throw away, recycle at charity shop. Both the latter two should be placed in black plastic bags. Once a decision has been made, it is important not to return to the decision again. This has been labelled as the "Only Handle It Once", or OHIO, principle by Randy Frost and Gail Steketee in their book.[1]

This activity of clearing should only continue for a maximum of 2 hours (maybe shorter depending on the individual). This is because it is almost impossible to fully concentrate for any longer than this. Sorting and clearing is a highly emotional and sometimes upsetting activity for the person to undertake and is extremely tiring due to this. Continuing to clear items while tired is more likely to result in mistakes. It is important to have breaks and rest so that the person can come back refreshed, but still a maximum of 2 hours is probably optimal. Once the clearing for the day has been done, the bags that are to be discarded should be removed from the property. For this reason, it is helpful to have someone helping with the sorting of items who can remove the bags to be discarded so that the person who has hoarding problems is not tempted to go and retrieve items later. To begin with, the person may ruminate about their decisions for a considerable time afterwards. If the items that have been discarded are easily accessible, then it is very tempting for the person to "rescue" them.

It is also important to remember that this sorting process is a marathon (or even an ultramarathon) and certainly not a sprint. Doing a regular 2-hour slot every day will soon make an impact and results should soon be apparent.

- **Rewarding yourself**

The work of clearing a living space and regaining the home is tiring and emotional. It is, therefore, important that the person who is doing this can reward themselves for their achievements. This could be as simple as "When I have cleared this chair, I am going to sit down and drink a cup of coffee in it". Or celebrating a bigger achievement, such as "When I have cleared the bathroom, I am going to have a long soak in a bubble bath". Once a room is completely cleared, rewards may be things like inviting a close family member home. In short, there should be many "rewards" scheduled into the process. These should be regular daily "rewards", such as sitting having a cup of coffee, and larger ones for even bigger achievements.

For some people who spent money on buying items or who spent large amounts of money on additional self-storage space, etc., tackling the hoarding may mean they have more money. Of course, many in these situations also may have debts which need to be addressed, but a small amount of money saved could be used for a special bath product or a nice cake from the tea shop!

Also, it is important to remember that clearing can take many months or even years. As the habit of sorting and discarding develops, so it becomes easier.

- **Relapse prevention**

Old habits can die hard, so it's important to ensure that the changes made during treatment translate into long-term changes and new more productive habits. Towards the end of clearing the hoard, making a relapse prevention plan is very important to prevent relapse. This means looking at issues which may make acquisition of items or failure to throw them away more likely. For example, we have already mentioned that going to a shopping centre when feeling miserable may make an impulse buy more likely. Similarly, if there is an urge to "save" certain items, it is best to avoid certain areas such as recycling points. Recognising the emotions which can lead to obtaining an item is also important. Sometimes people are diverted by their hoarding behaviours from addressing their problems of depression, loneliness, or isolation. Recognising these emotions and thinking of ways to address them can be vital in preventing relapse.

It can be hard for a person with hoarding to see past their hoarding behaviours, but now that their time is freer from the restraints of their hoarding they may be able to take up a new hobby or interest. This may be going to the local leisure centre for a swim, walking regularly or joining a walking group, joining a creative club, attending events in the local library, etc.

It is also important that the person looks out for signs that they are starting to hoard again. This requires the person to be brutally honest with themselves. Writing a list of warning signs can be very helpful. The key then is to start tackling the hoarding as soon as it arises and hopefully before it becomes a more major problem.

The case history of Carmen demonstrates many of the important points to remember in successful treatment.

Carmen's Story

Carmen is a 50-year-old woman who lives alone in a small flat in the city centre. She was born in the West Indies but moved to the UK as a baby with her mother, who worked in the National Health Service (NHS). When Carmen was 5 years old, her mother became very ill, and Carmen was sent back to the West Indies to live with her maternal grandmother. Whilst living with her grandmother, Carmen remembered this as a generally happy time but that she had few material possessions and would play with items she found outside.

When she was 11 years old, she was sent back to the UK to live with her mother. Carmen found this a very difficult time being taken away from the life she knew in the West Indies. In addition, she was bullied and made fun of at school due to her having a different accent to the other children, and she also experienced racism as her school was predominantly white. At this time, she remembered collecting things she thought were pretty such as the silver wrappers from a bar of chocolate. Knowing her mother would throw these away, she hid them in her room.

Leaving school at 16 years old without qualifications, Carmen started to work as a hospital cleaner and remained in this job until recently. She never married but did have a son who is now 32 years old as the result of a failed relationship. Her son, Milo, now lives in another part of the UK.

Two years ago, Carmen was diagnosed with breast cancer. Milo came to stay with her whilst she underwent surgery and started subsequent radiotherapy. On arriving at Carmen's flat, Milo was deeply shocked. Everywhere was covered with books, leaflets, plastic bags full of wrapping paper, and other paper and plastic items that Carmen had found or been given. He realised that the flat in the state it was in was unsuitable for Carmen to return to after her treatment.

He told his mother that he would arrange to get someone to come in and help him clear the flat. Carmen then became very upset and tearful, saying that she could not allow this to happen and that she needed all the items in the flat. Milo tried to argue with her but when he did so, Carmen insisted that if she needed to throw away her possessions, she would refuse to go into hospital and refuse to have treatment for her cancer. Milo could not understand her reluctance and the vehemence of her protests and went to visit Carmen's general practitioner (GP). When Milo had been growing up, Carmen had always had the tendency to hoard items that other people might throw away, but this had never got completely out of hand. Milo remembered that he always noticed that his house was fuller of plastic bags and items than any of his friends' homes. He suspected that the problem had grown since he left home to work 12 years ago. The GP listened to Milo's story and arranged for Carmen to be assessed by the local mental health service. In the meantime, Milo spoke with his mother, and she agreed that he could move some of the plastic bags into the attic provided he promised not to throw anything away. Milo moved plastic bags sufficient so that Carmen could get to the cooker and there was no fire risk, could have a bath, sit on the sofa, and sleep in her bed.

After her surgery, Carmen returned home. A therapist from the mental health unit asked to visit her at home. To begin with, Carmen was very reluctant to agree to this. Milo promised her that he would stay with her while the therapist visited and explained to Carmen that these were people who were very used to visiting people who might have cluttered homes. Carmen was still ashamed and embarrassed but agreed to meet the therapist.

The therapist was a young woman named Sue. She explained to Carmen and Milo that she worked in the local mental health team and had a special interest in working with people with hoarding issues. Explaining that she was far from shocked by Carmen's flat and that she had been in many more-cluttered environments, Sue also reassured Carmen that she was not going to throw away any of her possessions, but that Carmen herself would be in control of the therapy.

Sue then took a detailed history from Carmen and Milo. After an hour, Sue said,

"Thank-you for telling me your story. It seems that you have a condition known as Hoarding Disorder. This is a very common condition, and you can be helped to live in a more comfortable home. People hoard items for a variety of reasons. From what you have told me it seems that you had few possessions in your early life. We know that people who grow up in environments where they have few possessions may be more prone to hoard later in life. When you returned to the UK, you were moved into a very different situation, and in addition, you were bullied. We know that adversity like this can also make it more likely that people hoard possessions. In your case, you "escaped" from the bullying and racism by keeping some pretty items which you cherished.

Once Milo was born you were extremely busy being a single mother and also holding down a full-time job which was stressful. Although you may still have collected items at this time, it was more under control.

When Milo left home, there was an increased tendency to collect more items. You were living alone and didn't have any friends and, inevitably, missed your son. This has meant that your hoarding has now increased, and it is difficult for you to use your home in the way you would like. As you have been a cleaner all your life, you like to keep things clean and tidy; but, by having too many possessions, this has become impossible. In addition, you recently were made redundant from work, as the Hospital Trust you worked for retendered their cleaning services. This was a huge stress after all these years and would add to your tendency to hoard. Finally, you have had to come to terms with this diagnosis of cancer, which would also be a huge stress for you."

Sue went on to explain how most, but not all, people with Hoarding Disorder have a predisposition to develop the disorder and a family member who may have or did have similar issues. Carmen remembered that her great uncle in the West Indies had collected huge amounts of tree branches until no one could get into his garden. Sue explained about how certain events and situations can predispose someone to develop Hoarding Disorder. In addition, there may be precipitating factors to make this develop and finally current situations which make the hoarding continue despite a less than ideal living situation and which they labelled as "perpetuation factors". They then drew the following table of Carmen's Hoarding Disorder.

Table 8.1 How Carmen's Hoarding Disorder has developed

Predisposing factors	Precipitating factors	Perpetuating factors (what keeps the behaviour going)
Family history of hoarding in the family	Moving to the UK and to an alien environment alone	Loneliness and isolation
Few material possessions in childhood	Bullied at school	Being made redundant
	Living alone since Milo left home	Cancer diagnosis

Once this was drawn out, everyone could see that there were many reasons for Carmen having a hoarding problem. Sue then went on to explain that there was help that Carmen could receive and that she believed that, if she wished to really do this, she would do very well. It was agreed that Sue would return next week and discuss more fully what treatment would involve. In the meantime, Sue asked if Carmen would let her take some photographs on her phone of each of the rooms in the flat. Carmen was suspicious and unwilling at first, but Sue explained that these were purely for their records so that, when she progressed in treatment, they could look at where they had started. This was agreed and Sue took some photographs. It was also agreed by Carmen that no new items would come into the flat from now on and until the end of treatment. Although she was apprehensive about her ability to comply with this request, Carmen could see that it made sense and agreed to give it a try. Sue reassured her that everyone does slip up from time to time and that is not a big issue. The important thing is that, if you do slip up, you realise this and start to try to comply again. It was explained that many people use small slip-ups in their plan to say that they are unable to do this, but it is totally normal for people to have these slip-ups from time to time. Sue explained that, in some ways, a slip-up is good as it allows you to learn how to cope with these situations in the future without allowing yourself to go back to square one!

The following week, Carmen was on her own as Milo had returned home. She was extremely anxious and worried about what Sue might be planning for them to do. As agreed the previous week, Carmen had decided that her priority would be to start by clearing the living room. Sue arrived and suggested that they start by taking one of the bags in the living room. Asked what the chosen bag contained, Carmen said it was silver paper wrappers and leaflets. Sue then asked if Carmen would be prepared to throw this away. At this point, Carmen became tearful and said that this would be impossible as the things inside were so pretty. Sue agreed to halt proceedings and, asking Carmen to put the bag down, they started to look at Carmen's thoughts concerning this. The conversation is shown below:

SUE: "What are you thinking at the moment?"

CARMEN: "I'm scared you are going to ask me to throw away this bag and I will never see it again."

SUE: "I am not going to force you to do anything you do not want to but I would like to look at your thoughts concerning this. What would be so bad about losing this one bag which is one of many hundreds of similar ones which you have in the flat?"

CARMEN: "I really love pretty things and these things are pretty. I want to keep them so that I can have these pretty things in my life."

SUE: "I can understand that, but I wonder what the effect is of having so many bags of pretty things in your flat?"

CARMEN: "I guess it means that I can't use the flat as I should, and the whole place looks a mess. I'm embarrassed to invite friends to visit me here."

SUE: "Is it possible that, if you were to clear some of these bags, you could make the living room a pretty place and use a few of the contents of the bags that you really like to really make the place pretty?"

CARMEN: "I suppose at the moment I really can't see the pretty things I own."

SUE: "Yes that's right. Let's take this bag and go through it and I want you to decide what you really want to keep and what

I can take away with me. I want you to make an immediate decision, and I don't want you to hold any item for more than a few seconds. I also want you to agree that once the decision is made, then this is final, and there's no going back and changing your mind as we have to move forward."

Carmen reluctantly agreed with this, and over the course of the 2-hour session, managed to empty several bags with Sue taking away two big black rubbish sacks full of things to throw away. Carmen's immediate reaction was to be pleased with the progress she had made, and she could see that there was now a clear area just next to the sofa.

After Sue left, however, Carmen became very upset and started crying uncontrollably about what she had "lost". The next morning, she telephoned Sue, and after begging her to return the items, she said she no longer wanted to do the therapy. Sue talked to her on the phone, and they set up another meeting to talk rather than continue to clear the house. Carmen agreed when Sue asked even if she was not going to continue in therapy, would she agree to not bring any new items into the house until she had met with her.

At the next session, Carmen and Sue looked at Carmen's thoughts concerning her possessions. It became clear to both of them that Carmen had had a deprived upbringing with few possessions, and then when she had been bullied, she had taken solace from surrounding herself with pretty things. She had convinced herself as a child that, if she had these pretty things, she would become attractive to others who would be attracted by her "pretty things". As they started to examine these beliefs, Carmen could see that this was a child's answer to unhappiness but was not based in reality. Having so many piles of bags of pretty things not only meant that could Carmen not appreciate them but also it prevented her having friends as she was too ashamed to invite people home. In other words, something that was supposed to attract people to her was actually having the opposite effect.

At the end of the session, Carmen agreed to continue a clearing session with Sue the next week.

Therapy continued for the next 6 weeks, and Carmen was able to clear the rest of the living room. They had some minor problems when Carmen became upset, but she was getting better at challenging her distressing thoughts and was starting to feel pleased with her progress. At the beginning of therapy, it had been agreed that she would "treat" herself after achieving a milestone. Carmen chose to go out and buy herself a really pretty mirror to hang on the living room wall. She was so delighted with her room and felt she now might be able to invite someone in for a coffee.

Towards the end of the 6 weeks, Sue had introduced Carmen to Lucy, who was a peer-support worker who was attached to the mental health unit in the Trust. Lucy would be able to continue working with Carmen for several more weeks until the whole flat was cleared, and Carmen would just see Sue once a month at the community mental health service base to ensure everything was continuing to go well.

Three months later Carmen did manage to complete her treatment and now has a lovely tidy flat that she can clean and keep tidy. She has invited old colleagues from the hospital to the flat and has had not just Milo but also his girlfriend to stay with her. Milo is so very proud of his mum and her achievements. Although Carmen worries that she may slip up and go back, she has written a relapse prevention plan which she keeps next to her bed to remind her of the danger. The relapse plan looks like this:

Signs I may be relapsing

- Finding myself putting wrappers to one side
- Collecting a bag full of scraps
- Feeling low and miserable

What I need to do if I am relapsing

- Resist and throw away the items before they start to overwhelm me
- Reach out to friends for support
- Take myself out for a coffee, have a long soak in the bath, or wash my hair/do my makeup to make myself feel better

The story of Carmen shows that treatment can be a lengthy process but that it is not important how long it takes as long as overall things are moving forwards.

Carmen had individual treatment, but sometimes another type of approach in the form of group treatment can be useful.

Individual versus Group CBT

It is not uncommon to be offered group treatment for hoarding. There has been plenty of research on this option, and in general it seems to work equally as well, or in some reports better, than individual treatment. There are obviously some advantages as well as disadvantages to receiving group treatment rather than individual therapy.

- **Disadvantages**
  - You may have to wait until a group is ready to start, but there is often a long (or even longer) wait for individual therapy.
  - You receive less individualised time with a therapist.
  - You need to commit to a certain time frame and to attending therapy meetings on a regular basis (this is also true of individual therapy, but when there is just one person involved, there may be greater flexibility).
  - It can feel as if not all the sessions are applicable to your particular issues.
  - If you have been isolated for a length of time, meeting a group can seem extremely daunting.

- **Advantages**
  - Being in a group of people with similar problems can be reassuring and make individuals feel less "alone" in suffering from this condition.
  - Other group members share their own experiences and help each other with support and also ideas for overcoming obstacles.
  - As everyone in the group has similar issues, the shame and stigma many people with Hoarding Disorder feel is not present in the group.
  - People with similar problems can often be much more helpful in describing their lived experience rather than the experience of

professionals, which is usually learned from observation, talking, and books.

o The group often can forge friendships which exist outside of the group therapy sessions and last well after therapy ends. These friends can support each other and point out if they feel things are going wrong.

o The rate of people dropping out of treatment for Hoarding Disorder is relatively high and estimated in research studies to be between 20 and 50 per cent for individual therapy and between 10 and 40 per cent for group treatment. It has been reported anecdotally that people may be less inclined to drop out of a group than individual therapy as they do not wish to disappoint the group or let them down. Also, the informal support networks which often grow amongst the group members may reduce the tendency to drop out. In other words, if you are feeling like dropping out of treatment but a friend calls you and encourages you not to, maybe with stories of how they have felt in a similar situation, you may be less inclined to give in.

o Not everyone always gets along with everyone. In individual therapy, if you don't get along with your therapist, it can be very difficult. With a group situation, you are more likely to find some people you do like as well as the risk that you may not get along with everyone in the group.

From the point of view of provision of services, clearly it may be more cost-efficient to have people being treated in a group rather than individually. For this reason alone, I suspect increasing numbers of people will be likely to be offered group rather than individual therapy in the future. As noted earlier, studies have estimated that between 2 and 5 per cent of the population have significant hoarding. If we take the lower figure of 2 per cent and look at what that means in the UK with a population of approximately 67 million people, then 1,340,000 people in the UK are likely to have significant hoarding issues. As we have seen, group therapy can be at least as effective as individual treatment and may have some additional benefits as well.

Compassion Focussed Therapy (CFT)

We have mentioned that many people with Hoarding Disorder drop out of treatment for their problems. We have also noted that many people with Hoarding Disorder experience intense shame, embarrassment, and stigma concerning their hoarding behaviours. CFT is a form of therapy which aims to address the shame and embarrassment many people experience when addressing their thoughts and emotions in CBT. It has been shown that, when compassion-focussed methods are added into a CBT programme, better outcomes and more improvements have been found in people with conditions such as depression, eating disorders, post-traumatic stress disorders, personality disorders, and psychosis. The emotional arousal and the shame associated with Hoarding Disorder and how these emotions may actually increase in some situations when tackling their problems using more standard CBT led some researchers and therapists to wonder if adding CFT to treatment packages with CBT might help to address this. So far there have been very few studies examining this issue. One recent but very small study did show that fewer people seemed to drop out of CFT and that they showed improvements in their condition.[2]

CFT has some distinct differences from traditional CBT. Firstly, it examines our emotions in their evolutionary terms. Before modern civilisation, many resources were scarce and people would store and collect items for future use. This was mentioned in the first chapter when we described how many animals hoard to see them through the winter. Similarly, humans would preserve and store food but also other possessions which could be used in the future. The natural urge to save and collect is, therefore, deeply rooted in our brains. In our modern civilisation, we have limited living space compared to the whole natural environment, and also do not need to store up items when we have multiple shops as well as online stores which can supply our every need. In CFT, the natural instinctive need to hoard is recognised and used to explain the current hoarding behaviour.

Secondly, during therapy with CFT, people undergoing treatment are encouraged to identify their unpleasant emotions and recognise how they arise deep in the brain and are not anyone's "fault" but a natural process that was helpful to our ancestors' survival.

Mindfulness is used in CFT to reduce the critical self-talk often experienced by people with Hoarding Disorder. Based on Eastern concepts of meditation, mindfulness teaches individuals to let their thoughts and emotions happen, recognise them for what they are without self-judgement, and accept that they will occur but that they do not matter in the process. In addition, focussing on the present is a mindfulness technique which can help a person with hoarding to decide whether to discard or keep a particular item.

During the process of CFT, the therapist works with the person with hoarding problems to develop self-soothing techniques which can be used in a variety of situations to reduce the impact of the upsetting emotions which arise.

Although the techniques of CFT do appear promising for Hoarding Disorder, there is not sufficient research to wholeheartedly recommend it for everyone at this time. Some of the techniques, such as adopting a non-judgemental attitude towards yourself and recognising deep-seated emotions for what they are, rather than responding to the emotions as if they are reality, can be usefully incorporated into treatment for everyone.

KEY POINTS

- CBT is the main psychological treatment which is useful for Hoarding Disorder.
- CBT for Hoarding Disorder involves:
  - Education about the condition and treatment
  - Agreement to stop new items entering the property
  - Learning to organise, sort, and discard items
  - Rewarding oneself
  - Relapse prevention

- Hoarding treatment groups have been shown to be as effective as individual treatment and may offer some additional benefits for some people.
- Dropout from treatment for Hoarding Disorder is common, and techniques such as CFT are being examined to see if they successfully address this problem.

9

• • • • • • •

What About the Law and Hoarding?

Different countries, states, and provinces have different laws and legal systems. Laws also change with time. There are nevertheless some common threads regarding laws which affect hoarding and what may be your legal rights. In this chapter, we will start by examining the various laws which may be relevant for people who hoard in England, Wales, and much of the UK. We will then outline the differences from these laws in Scotland and Northern Ireland. Finally, we will mention how hoarding laws vary in Europe and the European Union, Australia, Canada, India, New Zealand, and the United States of America

Please note that we are not lawyers, and this chapter is meant to be an overview of our understanding of the law as it currently stands. It is aimed at providing a very approximate view of a person's rights. With any legal issues you or your family may experience, you are strongly advised to consult a solicitor for any legal advice.

In England and Wales, the main laws which may be applied fall under 10 possible Acts, which are:

- Mental Health Act 1983
- Mental Capacity Act 2005
- Children Act 1989
- Animal Welfare Act 2006
- Care Act 2014
- Public Health Act 1936
- Anti-Social Behaviour, Crime and Policing Act 2014
- Environmental Protection Act 1990
- Prevention of Damage by Pests Act 1949
- Housing Act 2004

Mental Health Act 1983

The Mental Health Act makes provision for the admission to hospital or other intervention, even against that person's wishes, if they are deemed to be suffering from a mental disorder and are believed to be either a danger to themselves or a danger to others. This Act can be applied in the community. The main sections of this Act which are likely to apply to people with hoarding issues are Section 2 and Section 3.

Section 2 of the Act requires two registered doctors, one of whom should have prior knowledge of the patient, and at least one of whom has specialised expertise in the diagnosis and treatment of mental disorders, to apply for an individual to be moved to a place of safety, for example, a hospital to protect their safety or the safety of other people. The doctors involved in this recommendation need to complete the following:

- **Assessment**. Thorough assessment of the person and assessment of their risk to themselves and others.
- **Diagnosis**. Although this is not mandatory or even sometimes possible at this stage, a diagnosis can help to inform the process.

- **Recommendation**. Based on the assessment the two doctors make, a recommendation regarding whether the individual is suffering from a mental illness and whether, as a result of mental illness or impairment, they are currently in a situation which means they are a risk to themselves or to other people. This recommendation is then passed to the social worker.
- **Ongoing care**. Usually, the doctor who knows the patient (very often a general practitioner [GP]) will be involved in planning future care after any hospitalisation.

Once the Section papers have been signed, they are reviewed, usually by a social worker, who liaises with the person and their next-of-kin to ensure that no alternative option can be applied and achieve the safety required. Other possible options may be the person moving temporarily to live with a relative, which they would do voluntarily. The social worker's job in this situation is:

- **Assessment**. Independently of the two medical recommendations, the social worker makes a thorough assessment of the individual, their risks, and needs.
- **Recommendation**. Based on their assessment, the views of the person and their relatives, the social worker makes a recommendation whether hospital admission is necessary or whether alternatives could be used.
- **Safeguarding**. The social worker needs to ensure that the person's rights are upheld. They will explain these rights to the person and their family.
- **Advocacy**. It is the role of the social worker to make sure the views of the person and their relatives are heard and taken into consideration in any care planning.
- **Care planning**. Care planning involves the team of psychiatrists, nurses, the social worker, and general practitioner to ensure appropriate help and care is put into place in both the present and future planning.

Section 2 provides for the individual to remain in hospital for up to 28 days, although the individual can appeal this decision to a Mental Health Tribunal within the first 14 days of being in hospital. The Mental Health Tribunal is a body, independent of the hospital, that assesses whether the law has been correctly applied and whether there are grounds for detaining an individual. They can also ask the hospital managers for a review of the decision at any point. In both of these situations, the person who is detained can ask for legal advice and representation from a solicitor or from an advocate. Most mental health hospitals in the NHS have an independent Advocacy Department that is experienced in these procedures.

Section 2 of the Mental Health Act is for observation, diagnosis, and to try to alter the situation so that the person can be discharged safely. It lasts for up to 28 days. If a person needs more than 28 days, then it is usual for the hospital to apply for Section 3, which lasts up to 6 months. This is similar in many ways to Section 2 except it is a "treatment order", during which patients are admitted for treatment rather than assessment and diagnosis as with Section 2. This section can also be appealed to a Tribunal or review requested to hospital managers.

The real-life story of Juanita demonstrates some aspects of the Mental Health Act.

Juanita's Story

Juanita is a 40-year-old lady who works in finance. She has suffered from prolonged periods of depression throughout her adult life. In the past, she had also experienced some brief periods when she had been elated but these had been controlled and had not required treatment.

Last year, she was promoted at work. Her job was a demanding one, and this new promotion meant that she was working extremely long hours. Around this time, she began spending more money on clothes and items for the home as she felt she deserved these to make up for her long hours at work. Her family and friends were concerned about her extremely long hours, but she dismissed their concerns, saying that she was coping.

She had always been a popular member of the work team, but it was noticed that Juanita would become snappy and uncharacteristically rude to colleagues. She then started to go out during the working day for prolonged periods and would become irritated and verbally abusive if this was mentioned. People also noticed that she started wearing increasingly unusual, brightly coloured clothes, many of which appeared unusual in a work setting, as well as wearing uncharacteristically bright make-up. Her managers became concerned and spoke with her sister about their concerns. Juanita was furious and insisted she was being victimised. She said that she had decided that, having reached the age of 40, she wanted to branch out more in her tastes and appearance. Her sister remained concerned but felt powerless to do more as she felt she had little evidence of any other issues. Despite this, her sister telephoned Juanita's key worker to express her concerns, and it was agreed that they would watch out for any deterioration.

In December last year, Juanita was arrested in a large high-end department store for shoplifting. She was found to have tried to take several items including dresses and handbags and was walking out of the store. When apprehended, Juanita became very angry and was insisting that she "had a right" to these items, claiming that she was the owner of the store. The police took her to the local mental health assessment unit under Section 136 of the Mental Health Act. This act gives the police the right to detain someone and take them to a place of safety for a mental health assessment if they believe the person is suffering a mental health crisis.

Juanita was assessed and thought to be in a hypomanic state, and it was decided that she needed to remain in hospital for further assessment. She was very distressed initially by being kept in hospital. However, as she began to settle and to receive help and treatment, she began to trust the staff more. Her sister was asked to bring some items from Juanita's home. On opening the door to the flat, her sister was horrified by the state of everything. Rubbish had not been cleared for several months, there were piles of possessions everywhere, including expensive-looking clothes and items on every surface. Indeed, it was clear that Juanita could only sleep on a small part of her bed as it was otherwise piled high with clothes. On the floor were piles of bills including demands for payments which were long overdue.

It was clear that Juanita had been spending large amounts of money, far more than she could afford, for many months. In addition, she had not done any cleaning or housework and had ignored her mail for a similar amount of time. When this was discussed with Juanita, she was very upset and said that she owed several thousand pounds which she could not pay. Her team asked the social worker attached to the hospital to visit Juanita and to look at how she might be able to handle her bills. It was also arranged for her to go home with her care coordinator to start sorting the flat, throwing out rubbish, etc. Some of the clothes in the property were new, unworn, and still had labels on them so could be returned for a refund, but the bulk had been worn or soiled. Juanita decided she would try and sell some of these clothes online to reduce the amount of money she owed. Arrangements were made for her to reduce the debts she had accrued on credit cards by taking out a bank loan which would be paid back over many months but at a lower rate of interest than the credit cards.

The story of Juanita demonstrates that, although sounding extremely frightening, application of the Mental Health Act can be a useful turning point for some individuals.

In Juanita's case, she had a history of Bipolar Disorder. Since 2013, Hoarding Disorder has been recognised as a mental disorder in its own right. It is difficult to know how many people with Hoarding Disorder, as opposed to the symptom of hoarding, are admitted under the Mental Health Act at this present time. However, everyone with a mental health issue should be entitled to the help and support they require.

Mental Capacity Act 2005

The Mental Capacity Act is different from the Mental Health Act in that it refers to an individual and their ability to make decisions regarding their care at a given point of time, which may be something that rapidly changes or stays fairly constant. Most people are considered to have capacity unless it can clearly be demonstrated otherwise. The Mental Capacity Act is not used to restrict decision making in those who are fully able to make a decision and cannot be used to prevent someone making an unwise decision if they have full capacity. For example, I may decide to take a sugar pill rather than receive the treatment needed for cancer. If I meet the criteria for full capacity, however unwise my decision is, no one can prevent me from making this decision. Mental capacity may be impaired either constantly or from time to time by:

- Mental illness of various types
- Dementia
- Learning disability
- Substance misuse
- Delirium, confusion, drowsiness, or unconsciousness due to illness or treatment of this illness

If the Mental Capacity Act is to be applied, it needs to be shown that every help and assistance has been provided to help them make that decision. It applies to people aged 16 years and older living in England and Wales.

If a person is deemed not to have capacity, then other people may be required to make a decision for them. This may be:

- A person granted Lasting Power of Attorney (LPA) by the individual when they had capacity. There are two types of LPA. One is for welfare and health decisions and the second for financial and property decisions.
- If there is no one with LPA, then the Court of Protection can appoint a Deputy to make decisions. This may be a family member, friend, or professional appointed by the court.
- Independent Mental Capacity Advocate (IMCA). The use of an IMCA is usually when there are no family and friends available and decisions need to be made about medical treatment or a change in accommodation. The IMCA is often a professional social worker or similar.

In order to assess someone's capacity, the following questions need to be addressed by the person making the assessment:

Is the person able to make the decision (with or without support)?

- If unable to make the decision, is there a disturbance in functioning of mind or brain?
- Is the inability to make the decision due to this disturbance of mind or brain?

The tests for whether or not they have the capacity to make the decision require that the person:

- Can understand the information given to them (with support if necessary).
- Remember and retain this information long enough to make the decision.
- Weigh up the information in order to make the decision.
- Communicate this decision to others either by talking or by sign language, or even by other means such as blinking the eyes when asked.

These tests should be completed at every capacity assessment. As previously mentioned, capacity can be a very temporary thing which fluctuates depending on the decision. The story of Pete illustrates this.

Pete's Story

Pete is a 50-year-old man with a history of OCD as well as Hoarding Disorder. He had voluntarily been admitted to a psychiatric ward to treat his OCD, which had not responded to attempts to treatment at home. He was doing well in his treatment of his OCD, which consisted of unpleasant and violent intrusive thoughts that distressed him greatly and caused him to perform anxiety-reducing compulsions of excessive showering and hand-washing to try and "wipe out" the thoughts. He lived with his wife and two teenaged sons in a house in a small town. Periodically, Pete would get very annoyed with his wife when she cleared out some of the possessions Pete accumulated in every part of the house and garden.

In hospital, the staff noticed that Pete's bedroom was becoming very cluttered. At first, they made a joke about it with him, and he agreed to tidy the room. However, it became worse and worse. Pete would go out every day for a long walk and would collect anything he found on his walks. These items included leaves, sticks, stones, and bits of detritus which he found down on the river bank. These items were put into plastic bags and stored in his room.

The staff spoke to Pete and explained the bags were damp and smelly and needed to be disposed of. Pete was insistent that they were important and that he needed to keep them. Any discussion was fruitless, and Pete refused to hand over any of his bags.

The staff felt that these bags were becoming hazardous. Pete had full mental capacity in almost all areas, but in regards to his bags of rubbish, he was unable to weigh up the evidence in favour of disposing of the bags, as his Hoarding Disorder meant he was not able to make a fully rational decision. The staff then removed some of these items from Pete's room, giving him the option to work with them, which he refused. The bags were removed as it was felt to be in Pete's best interest to remove these bags of rotting leaves and papers.

Pete was extremely upset at losing his bags but over the next few weeks agreed to work with the staff on tackling his Hoarding Disorder as well as his OCD.

Children Act 1989

This Act sets out the legal framework for the protection and welfare of children in the UK. A child should live in a home with space to play and function, not be at risk of harm, and be able to invite friends home. In the case of children, it is always advisable to act on the side of caution and intervene early.

Schools, social services, and national charities, such as the National Society for the Prevention of Cruelty to Children (NSPCC), can offer help, advice, and assessment if there are any concerns.

The concern of parents is always that their children may be removed from them. In reality, this is always the very last resort and is not a decision which is taken lightly. It is much more common for help and support to enable the family to stay together and to cope better to be offered.

Animal Welfare Act 2006

This Act applies to people who are hoarding animals as discussed in Chapter 4. However, it also applies to people who live in a hoarded home which is unsuitable for housing an animal. Under the Animal Welfare Act, an animal must be fed and watered and allowed sufficient space to carry out its natural activities. It should also be kept in a hygienic environment. As discussed in Chapter 4, animal charities such as the Royal Society for the Prevention of Cruelty to Animals (RSPCA) have the powers to intervene and even remove animals if they find the animal is suffering. In reality, the RSPCA will normally try and find a solution in collaboration with the owner and are generally reluctant to seize animals unless really necessary.

Care Act 2014

The Care Act is primarily involved with ensuring that individuals receive the support and care that they need. It does not specifically target hoarding, but if someone is living in a severely hoarded environment, then the local authority should assess what care and support may be needed to help this person.

Public Health Act 1936

This Act gives the local authorities power to intervene if an individual is hoarding materials which make the environment unsafe or dangerous to other people in the area, such as a risk of fire in a block of flats or toxic or unhygienic items in communal areas or adjacent to other people.

Anti-Social Behaviour, Crime and Policing Act 2014

This Act has only occasional relevance to hoarding. Under this Act, local authorities and police have powers to address anti-social behaviour, which may include hoarding if this impacts on the local community or is a risk to health and safety.

Local authorities can issue Community Protection Notices where the individual is told to clean up the hoard or face criminal prosecution. The police can apply for closure orders whereby they may order the closure of a building or space that was deemed to be causing a public nuisance.

Finally, local authorities could issue a Public Spaces Protection Order if the hoarding behaviour is impacting on public areas.

Environmental Protection Act 1990

This Act may occasionally be applied in hoarding situations. Firstly, with the issue of duty of care, whereby waste, including that from hoarding, must be properly managed and disposed of.

If the hoarding is considered to cause a statutory nuisance by virtue of smells, vermin, or other public health issues, then local authorities can insist that the problem is solved and the offending items and hoard removed.

Prevention of Damage by Pests Act 1949

Local authorities have the powers to take control of pests which may thrive in a hoarded environment.

Housing Act 2004

If a hoarding problem is causing a risk to other inhabitants' properties such as structural damage due to weight of hoarded items in a block of flats or obstructing exits with risk of fire and falls, etc., then the local authorities can take action to address these hazards.

As can be seen from the above, there are several laws which may be applied to hoarding in England and Wales. There are some differences in other countries in the UK, but overall, the same principles apply, as shown in Table 9.1, which also addresses some of the relevant legislation in other countries in the world.

Table 9.1 Laws which may be applied to hoarding

Country or region	Laws
Scotland	• Mental health legislation = Mental Health Care and Treatment Act 2003. • Adult Support and Protection (Scotland) 2007 Act = same as Care Act. • Children (Scotland) Act 1995. • Housing Scotland Act 2006. • Local authority powers are similar in Scotland and England and Wales.
Northern Ireland	• Mental Health (Northern Ireland) Order 1986. • Adult Safeguarding (Northern Ireland) Order 2015. • Children (Northern Ireland) Order 1995. • Housing (Northern Ireland) Order 2003 = safety of housing. • Local authority powers similar to England and Wales.
Europe and the EU	It is impossible to summarise the various laws which may be used in hoarding in a variety of countries with different legal systems. In the main, they are broadly similar to those described in the UK. For example, in Spain, hoarding is regarded as a mental health issue and is covered by the Mental Health Act (Ley de Salud Mental), which means that people with hoarding have the right to receive appropriate care, help, and treatment. Another law is the Law on Urban Leases (Ley de Arrendamientos Urbanos), which allows a landlord to terminate a lease if a tenant is excessively hoarding. Also in Spain, local municipalities have laws regarding public health and safety with respect to hoarding behaviour.
Australia	Each state and territory in Australia has its own mental health legislation. These laws govern the assessment, treatment, and care of individuals with mental health problems, including Hoarding Disorder. These laws include those similar to the Mental Health Act in England and Wales. Other laws include: Child Protection Acts (each state and territory in Australia has its own Child Protection Acts).

Table 9.1 (Cont.)

Country or region	Laws
	Residential tenancy legislation. Local government regulations. Public health legislation.
Canada	Mental health legislation: Each province and territory in Canada has its own mental health legislation. Child and Family Services Act. Housing legislation in Canada is primarily regulated at the provincial and territorial levels. Fire and building codes in Canada are typically established at the provincial and territorial levels. Public health legislation in Canada is also regulated at the provincial and territorial levels.
India	Mental Healthcare Act 2017: Comprehensive mental health legislation. Juvenile Justice (Care and Protection of Children) Act 2015. Building codes cover structure and safety of living areas. Each state in India has its own public health act that addresses issues related to sanitation, cleanliness, and public health hazards.
New Zealand	Mental Health (Compulsory Assessment and Treatment) Act 1992. Oranga Tamariki Act 1989. Health and Safety at Work Act 2015. Building Act 2004.
United States of America	Mental health laws in the USA vary across states with each state having its own specific laws regarding assessment and treatment of those with mental ill health. There are also some federal laws such as the Mental Health Parity and Addiction Equity Act (2008), which requires insurance plans to provide equal coverage for mental and addiction health issues as they do for physical disorders. Child protective services laws: these differ from state to state but are aimed at ensuring the welfare of children. Building and fire codes are locally governed.

Country or region	Laws
	Many cities and states have housing codes which describe the minimum standards for the condition and maintenance of residential properties.
	Nuisance laws vary by jurisdiction, but they may cover issues related to hoarding.
	Some states have laws and agencies dedicated to protecting vulnerable adults, including those with hoarding disorders.

KEY POINTS

- There are various laws which may be applicable to hoarding. These vary across countries but mostly fall under certain categories. In this bulleted list are the main ones in England and Wales, but many countries have similar laws (as shown in Table 9.1).

- The Mental Health Act (1983) in England and Wales is the provision for a person with mental health problems, mental disability, or cognitive impairment to receive help and treatment, even against their will, if they are placing themselves or others in danger. Similar Acts exist in most countries.

- The Mental Capacity Act (2005) is different from the Mental Health Act as it recognises that people may be able to make decisions in some areas and not others and that sometimes people are unable to understand, retain, and weigh up evidence in respect to certain decisions. In these cases, decisions may need to be made for them in their best interest.

- The welfare of any children living in a hoarded property is of paramount importance. This is covered by the Children Act (1989).

- The Animal Welfare Act (2006) is designed to ensure that animals are kept in a suitable environment with sufficient space to move around and that it is hygienic.

- Other Acts include the Care Act (2014), Public Health Act (1936), Anti-Social Behaviour, Crime and Policing Act (2014), Environmental Protection Act (1990), Prevention of Damage by Pests Act (1949), Housing Act (2004).

10

· · · · · · ·

How Can Someone with Hoarding Disorder Help Themselves?

In this chapter, we examine how people with Hoarding Disorder can help themselves. This is not a "quick fix", and it does take time, commitment, and courage to face up to your problems. We will start by looking at how a ban on new items coming into the property is the first "golden rule" of treatment. We will examine how it can be useful but not essential to have a friend or family member also involved in the process. The principles of discarding objects are discussed with the idea of holding on to objects for the shortest time possible, making an immediate decision and then sticking with it and not going back on that decision. Finally, we will list helpful resources and groups who may be able to assist you.

Why Should I Change My Habits?

One of the toughest parts of starting to tackle hoarding is realising and admitting that you have a problem. If you live in a situation for a long time, you become accustomed to this situation and can be surprised when other people feel it could be a problem. As we have seen earlier in this book, there are many issues which can occur with hoarding which could place you or others around you in danger. The first important thing to do is to take a long hard look at your environment and try to imagine an outsider looking at your home. Then ask yourself the following questions:

- Would I really be happy to invite someone into my home without embarrassment?
- Can I find the things I cherish, or is it virtually impossible in the pile of objects everywhere?
- Can I properly clean my house, or do the piles of things make this impossible?
- Can I use the main rooms of my house for the purposes for which they are designed? (e.g., Can I cook safely with a cooker which is not surrounded by objects? Can I use the bathroom and toilet without stepping over objects? Can I sit and watch TV on the sofa with a cup of tea on the coffee table? Can I sleep in my bed without being surrounded by things?)
- Can I safely use all entrances and exits to my property without being impeded by or having to climb over objects?
- Can I use the heating system in my home, or is access to it blocked?
- Have I had issues with vermin (e.g., rats, mice, cockroaches, etc.)?
- Have I blocked communal entrances or used my garden/outside space to store items that will not fit in the house?
- Have I felt the need to rent extra storage space to accommodate my "collections"?

If you have answered "yes" to any of the above, then it is likely you may have a hoarding problem. The next things to think about are the advantages and disadvantages of remaining as you are as opposed to tackling the issue (assuming you are not being made to tackle it by an external agency such as the local council). The advantages and disadvantages vary from individual to individual, but it can be really helpful to set them out on a sheet of paper. An example and suggestions are given in Table 10.1.

Table 10.1 Advantages and disadvantages of remaining as you are

Disadvantages of remaining as I am	Advantages of remaining as I am
The house is crowded, and I am unable to really enjoy the space I have or use it fully.	This is familiar, and I've lived like this for many years.
I am embarrassed and feel humiliated as I know my house is messy.	Familiarity is comfort to me.
I am unable to put the heating on, and it is very cold in winter.	I know all my possessions are here in the house somewhere.
I am unable to cook a full meal in the kitchen.	It gives me satisfaction to think I have everything I need.
I am unable to have a bath/shower due to items in the bathroom.	It just feels too overwhelming to start to clear the items as there are just too many, and I do not want others handling my stuff and throwing it away.
I cannot use the back door to my property.	I love my possessions and would find it very hard and upsetting to part with them.
My neighbours/the council/my family are complaining about my living situation.	
I have tripped and fallen over my things.	
I have a problem with mice/rats/cockroaches, etc.	
My property is damp as I can't heat it and allow air circulation.	

Table 10.1 (Cont.)

Disadvantages of remaining as I am	Advantages of remaining as I am
I have been unwell due to repeated chest infections related to cold/damp/dust.	
I have accumulated bills from renting storage units/lockups.	
It would be lovely to be able to invite friends/family into my house, but I can't at present.	

Table 10.1 is not meant to be a full list, and not all of these issues will apply to everyone, but it is an example of the kind of things that may be important to someone with hoarding. Setting out the advantages and disadvantages in this way may help to clear your mind as to why it may be helpful to start to tackle your hoarding.

Of course, not everyone does want to clear their hoarded items, but they may be under pressure from others to do so. We have already seen how local authorities (Chapter 9) and others may insist that a property is cleared. If this happens, it can seem as if everyone is trying to upset and harm you and your way of living. In most cases, it is much better to start to tackle the issue before the local authorities or others become involved. Indeed, some people have found themselves facing eviction due to hoarding. Most people feel that it would be better to start tackling the issue before it reaches this stage.

Starting to Help Yourself: Goal Setting

When tackling any problem, it is a good idea to have a clear plan of what you want to ultimately achieve. It can therefore be helpful to set out overall goals as well as intermediate and short-term goals.

Long-term goals are where you would like to be at the end of this process. These will normally take 6 months or more to achieve. Examples of long-term goals are:

"To live in my property while being able to cook using the oven and hob in the kitchen, use the heating, sit on the sofa, sleep in bed, and use all aspects of the bathroom."

Or it may be a more personal goal such as:

"To be able to have my grandchildren to stay with me without worrying about them falling over items in my home."

Whatever the overall goal is, it is worthwhile writing down to remind yourself when you start treatment.

Next, move on to setting intermediate goals. These are goals which may take several weeks or a few months to achieve and may be things like:

"To clear my kitchen so that I can use all work surfaces and access the oven and hob without moving clutter each time."

"To clear the bathroom so that I can sit on the toilet, stand at the washbasin, and climb into the bath without standing on items."

"To be able to sleep in my bed with all my clothes in the wardrobe and without having to climb over piles of clothes on the floor."

"To sit in my living room and have a cup of tea (placing this on the coffee table) without having to move items, and to watch TV without having to move items which restrict my view."

"To clear my storage unit so that I am not paying high monthly fees for its rental."

You may have many intermediate goals, and indeed, someone may have all of the above. They are useful to document so that you can monitor when you have achieved this. Achieving a medium-term goal is a cause for a big celebration, it is important that you celebrate and congratulate yourself on what you have achieved! Setting out in advance of achieving an intermediate goal what "reward" you are working towards can help with motivation. Having a room to be proud of is a big reward in itself but if you can also think of other ways of rewarding yourself for your hard work then this can be useful. Examples may be taking the day away from clearing the property and going somewhere you would like to go, such as a walk in the countryside, a visit to the beach, or even treating yourself to a meal in a favourite restaurant.

Finally, and possibly the most important, are the short-term goals or goals you wish to achieve along the way. These will normally take a week or so to achieve. For example, if you decide that you will clear the living room first, you need to decide on one area first. This may be around the sofa. The goal for that week (approximately) could be to clear the sofa and the area immediately surrounding it so that you can sit on the sofa with your feet on the floor. Once you have achieved this goal, again it is important to recognise your hard work and reward yourself with a treat. This may be sitting watching your favourite TV programme or going out for a cup of coffee in a local café. You can write these weekly goals down every week (some may take less or more than a week but approximately 5–10 days) and the reward you will give yourself.

Rewarding yourself is really very important for people with Hoarding Disorder. It is very common for people with Hoarding Disorder to blame themselves for their condition. This can lead to feeling depressed as well as feelings of self-disgust and even self-loathing. It is so important to remember that hoarding is not a "lifestyle choice" but is a mental disorder for which you are no more responsible than someone with rheumatoid arthritis is to blame for their condition. You are not to blame and you should regularly remind yourself of this fact, as well as the fact that you have shown both incredible resourcefulness as well as bravery in deciding to tackle your problem. Sadly, some parts of society have not yet caught up with this fact and do not realise that Hoarding Disorder is a mental disorder which can run in families and can be triggered by a number of social and environmental issues and requires treatment. People with determination and bravery can and do get better! As society and the media catch up with the science of Hoarding Disorder, it is important that individuals who suffer from the crippling effects of it are not led into believing the myths surrounding it! In short, be kind to yourself, this is not your fault, and you are being very brave in facing up to your fears and problems.

Starting to Plan Your Therapy

One of the first things to decide is whether you have a trusted friend or family member who is prepared to help you in your clearing of your home. This needs to be someone who is supportive and non-judgemental and who will not do anything without your consent even if you will occasionally have "lively" debates about what should be kept and what can go. This person can be helpful for a few reasons. Firstly, it can be really helpful to have the support of someone close who you can talk to honestly and openly and express your fears and emotions. Then it can help to have someone who can help you make quick choices and can demonstrate to you how to do this and maybe also help you in decision making in the future by teaching you their decision-making skills. The person must be patient and kind and also have the time to do this. They do not have to be with you every time you are clearing, but if they come even a few times, this may be helpful.

If you do not have any suitable person, then do not worry, you can still get better. You may find it particularly helpful to join a self-help group for people with hoarding problems. This can be really helpful whether or not you also have an individual helping you. At the end of this chapter, we list some self-help groups and their contact details, but inevitably this is not comprehensive, and neither does it cover every country in the world. You may find groups local to you which offer help. Before joining any group, make sure they are a self-help group and not a commercial enterprise looking to charge you for "decluttering services" or similar. Also always ask about their outcomes and successes. Some self-help groups are full of people who have not changed despite being members for many years. Whereas it may be nice for the members to have each other and to have support, you need to ensure that any group you join is about change and not just supporting you in your current situation.

After you have decided whether or not to tackle the hoarding with a friend or alone, and have found a supportive group looking to help you change, the next decision is which room do you want to start in. It can be very tempting to flit from room to room and area to area, but this means it is extremely hard to see any results. Choosing one room and one specific area means you will be able to notice your hard work and improvements very quickly. The choice of where to start is determined by a number of factors. The most important factor guiding this decision is whether there is any area which needs to be cleared to ensure your safety or that of others. If there is, then it is vital that this area is chosen first. For example, any items close to naked flames and causing a fire risk in the kitchen must be tackled urgently. Apart from any danger, afterwards the decision is down to you, but it may be helpful to think about tackling an area which will give you increased comfort and some pleasure when you finish. Examples may be the bathroom, where you could luxuriate in a hot bath once the bathroom is cleared, or it may be the living room or bedroom. It is entirely up to you.

Having decided on which room, then pinpoint a specific area you are going to start working in. Once again, restricting yourself to working in one specific area means that you will be able to see your progress quicker than if you flit around the room doing a bit here and there.

You are now almost ready to start, but a little more planning can help. You will be sorting items to discard and keep and placing those you choose to discard into black plastic bags. It may be some things can go to charity shops. The important issue though is how are you going to remove the items from your property without having the temptation to change your mind and "rescue" the items you have just discarded? This is where having someone else helping you with the clearing can be useful, as they can remove the items immediately after your clearing session. It may be possible that a friend or acquaintance passes a charity shop on a regular basis and would remove the items for you. With disposing of rubbish too, it can be helpful if this is disposed of away from your home, but this may not be possible. In any case, it is important that all items are removed from the house after you have completed a clearing session, and this is worth planning in advance in some detail. Although you may convince yourself that you can be strong and resist the temptation to take things out of the discard bags, this can be much more difficult at times when you are feeling tired, upset, and emotional, or generally "under the weather", so it is important to think about this in advance and plan accordingly.

Health and Safety Issues

Having already considered the health and safety aspects when deciding which room to start tackling, it is also important to think about your health and safety as you start to clear. It is important to think about the following:

- **Are there items piled high so that if I disturb them, I am in danger of causing an "avalanche" effect and injuring myself?**

You need to consider this carefully. There have been too many tragic situations where people have been crushed, causing bad injuries, or in extreme cases death, from hoarded items falling on top of them. If in any doubt whether or not this applies to you, then it is really important that you seek help from the local authorities or your healthcare professional. Do not start to clear any items if the hoard is above your thighs at all, and even if not that high, it can still cause significant damage.

It will take bravery to admit your problem and seek help, but we really cannot stress strongly enough how important this is!

- **Will I have to climb on objects and risk a fall and injuring myself?**

Just as with the risk of "avalanche" of items, there may also be a risk of falling. Once again, make an honest appraisal of your situation and seek help as above if in doubt. It is far better to have someone tell you they do not think it is a risk than for you to suffer an accident!

- **Are any of the items stored toxic and do I need to think about that in terms of handling the material, and also are there any issues in its safe disposal?**

Certain chemicals, toxic or hazardous waste materials, including some old-style cleaning products, may need special treatment regarding handling and disposal. If in doubt, then it is important you check with local authorities.

- **Will I be at risk of disturbing vermin of any kind?**

Vermin may be happily living in a hoard but may become more of a problem to you and any neighbours once disturbed as you clear the hoard. If there is any concern or doubt about this, then contact a pest control expert.

- **Are the items very dusty? Do I have any health conditions that make this a problem?**

Hoarded items that have been there for a considerable amount of time are likely to be dusty. Disturbing these items is inevitably going to result in more dust in the air. This is likely to result in coughing and sneezing in most people but could be much more serious if you have a lung condition such as asthma, chronic bronchitis, or chronic obstructive airway disease.

Everyone is advised to wear a mask capable of reducing the dust in the air that you breathe (the type of masks used during the COVID pandemic should suffice in most cases, but you can also obtain masks from hardware stores designed for dusty environments).

If you have a lung condition, then it is important to discuss with your GP before starting to clear items. Your doctor may be able to prescribe extra inhalers or may feel, in some cases, that it is too risky for your health for you to proceed. Please listen to and heed this advice if given!

- **Are there rotting items that may mean there is a health issue?**

Everyone is advised to wear latex gloves or similar when handling hoarded items due to dust and general dirt which may have accumulated. In the case of any rotting items, make sure these are disposed of quickly, and make sure you do not touch your face with your hands without thoroughly washing them.

The above is not an exhaustive list of potential hazards but does cover some of the main concerns. It is important that you think through exactly what types of things are amongst your hoarded items and what the risks may be in your individual circumstances.

Starting to Clear the Area

Once you are ready to start clearing, remember to wear old clothes and wear latex gloves as it may be dusty, and you may even need a dust mask and safety eyewear if it is very dusty to prevent you coughing and sneezing. Remember that this isn't going to be easy, and it will make you anxious and will be tiring. It is so important to be kind to yourself and remind yourself frequently that this is not your fault and that you are being very brave in admitting to the problem and deciding to tackle it.

If the hoarded items include a large number of papers such as bills, letters, leaflets, etc., it is important to have a shredder so that you can dispose of items without the risk of giving away information to others from documents such as old bank statements. If you do not own a shredder, you may be able to borrow one (as well as friends or family members having one, some local libraries have "libraries of things" where you can borrow equipment for a nominal fee) or else buy one cheaply.

With your opaque plastic bag at the ready, start with the first items, deciding whether to keep or discard. Pick up the first item and immediately make a decision about whether to keep or discard. Do not think for too long, just go with your first reaction. Once you've made your decision to discard, place the item immediately into the bag for disposal. It is really important that you do not hold onto the item for too long, only a few seconds at most. The longer you hold onto an item, the more difficult it is going to be to discard it. Make an immediate decision. Do not go backwards and forwards in your decision, but try and make an immediate snap decision. Once this is done, put the item out of sight and move on to the next item. This should then continue for a *maximum of 2 hours* or shorter, depending on how tired you feel. It's important not to go on for so long that you become too tired and won't be able to continue the next day. Once you have finished the clearing for the day, remove the black plastic bags from the home, and as far away as it is possible for you to put them.

It will be tempting to go back and change your mind about the items you have decided to discard. This is inevitable and can be very upsetting. However, it is important that you do not go back. As already mentioned in Chapter 8 in the story of Carmen, it is important that any item is only handled once and that the decision is immediate. This quick decision making will be very hard to begin with as many people with Hoarding Disorder have practised for years not making decisions such as these and may be spending many hours ruminating over items and as a consequence building up a hoard of items.

Once you have finished your clearing for the day, maybe try and get away from the home for a while by going for a walk, or if you prefer, having a relaxing time in the bath or having a cup of tea. Just a little reward to yourself after the clearing can be really helpful, even on a daily basis. What you have just done has been very hard and you have achieved it!

What if I Make a Mistake and Throw Away Something I Later Need/Want?

This is usually the biggest fear of someone with Hoarding Disorder. It is this fear that has led to you being trapped in a home overcrowded with items and unable to use the home for your needs. Although it may not seem that this is the case, as long as we have access to food and water, we will survive and do not need much else, apart from clothes to keep us warm and decent! We do not need to have every possible item in the home and if we were to throw away something which we subsequently discover could have been useful, we will probably be able to borrow or replace the item fairly easily. For example, when clearing through a pile of papers and shredding them, I suddenly discovered that, by not paying proper attention, I had shredded my medical degree! This was not a disaster, and a brief telephone call plus a letter meant I had a replacement very quickly. The important point is that everyone makes a mistake like this sometimes, and it is not the end of the world. Items can be replaced if necessary.

Do Not Forget to Reward Yourself

We have repeated this several times as we feel it is so very important. You are tackling a difficult problem and are bravely facing up to your fear, so you need to reward yourself regularly. This does not need to be expensive. Just a small reward such as a cup of tea at the end of a clearing session. After a significant milestone such as clearing an entire room, a more substantial reward would be in order. You could use some of the money you have saved by not purchasing new items for a special treat such as new bath products to pamper yourself with, a cup of coffee in a coffee shop, or even a meal out.

How Long Will It Take to Clear My Home?

This is, of course an impossible question to answer and will depend on the size of your home and how much stuff there is to clear. In general, this is a slow process, and it is likely that it will take weeks or months to clear an entire home. There is no hurry; as long as you continue to move forward, you will get there in the end! Don't set yourself an unrealistic time-frame. Also bear in mind that there will be days when you just do not feel strong enough to tackle it, or that you are unwell. At each point, be kind to yourself. If in doubt about whether to continue one day when you don't feel well, ask yourself what you would advise a close friend or family member that was in the same position as you, and then apply this advice to yourself.

Final Thoughts

Good luck as you start on this quest to regain your living space. Huge congratulations for recognising your problem and for taking the courageous step of deciding to tackle it. Key points at the very end of the chapter summarise the contents of this chapter. We are now listing details of various self-help and support organisations and self-help books on this subject.

Organisations Which Can Help

Hoarding UK

National charity that can provide support, information, and resources for people and families affected by hoarding. As well as advice on treatment and decluttering, they also offer services such as advocacy, etc.

https://hoardinguk.org

OCD Action

National charity that provides help and information for individuals and families affected by Obsessive Compulsive and Related Disorders including Hoarding Disorder

https://ocdaction.org.uk
0300 636 5478

OCD UK

National charity that provides help and information for individuals and families affected by Obsessive Compulsive and Related Disorders including Hoarding Disorder

www.ocduk.org
01332 588112 (09:00 – 12:00pm)

TOP UK (Triumph over OCD and Phobia)

A national charity which has a number of self-help treatment groups for people with a variety of fears, OCD, and Hoarding Disorder. These self-help groups can be in person or on-line.

www.topuk.org/
01225 571740
07907 344669
info@topuk.org

Scottish Association for Mental Health (SAMH)

SAMH is the leading mental health charity in Scotland and can offer help and advice for those with Hoarding Disorder and their families. They provide counselling, peer support, and advocacy services.

www.samh.org.uk
0344 800 0550

Northern Ireland Association for Mental Health (NIAMH)

Similar to SAMH, they offer counselling, peer support, and advocacy services.

www.niamhwellbeing.org
028 9032 8474

Local Authorities

Some local authorities have dedicated teams that can offer advice and help to families of hoarders.

Mental Health Services

Mental health services offer treatment and help to individuals with hoarding problems.

Useful Telephone Number and Websites in the USA

Child Protective Services (CPS)

A governmental agency.

800-422-4453

National Association of Professional Organizers (NAPO)

An organisation that includes professional organisers that specialise in Hoarding Disorder.

National Centre for Hoarding and Cluttering (NCHC)

This is a specialist organisation that offers training, consultancy, and support for professionals and families dealing with Hoarding Disorder. There is information on their website.

Children's Mental Health Services

Contact your local mental health department.

Hoarding Task Forces

Some cities and counties have dedicated task forces.

Other Books on Hoarding

This includes a selection of books on the market. It is not comprehensive but is an example of some of the titles available. Inclusion in this list does not imply that we endorse the title, nor does the omission of a title imply we do not recommend it.

1.   **David Tolin, Randy O. Frost, and Gail Steketee (2007) Buried in Treasures: Help for Compulsive Acquiring, Saving, and Hoarding.**

New York, NY: Oxford University Press. This is a self-help book which is divided into three sections which focus on different aspects of hoarding, viz. an introduction to hoarding; practical steps to help declutter; and finally how to remain "on track".

2. **Randy O. Frost and Gail Steketee (2010) Stuff: Compulsive Hoarding and the Meaning of Things.** *New York, NY: Houghton-Mifflin Harcourt.* A self-help book aimed at better understanding some of the psychology of hoarding.

3. **Gail Steketee and Christina Bratiotis (2020) Hoarding: What Everyone Needs to Know.** *New York, NY: Oxford University Press.* This is a book aiming to describe and help the individual better understand hoarding and its treatment. This book may be particularly useful to a lay audience who deal with hoarding in their professional life, for example, firefighters, social workers, and housing officers.

4. **Satwant Singh, Margaret Hooper and Colin Jones (2015) Overcoming Hoarding: A Self-Help Guide Using Cognitive Behavioural Techniques.** *London: Robinson.* This book is part of the "Overcoming" series which publishes self-help books in the UK for predominantly a UK market. Many of these titles have been placed on the "Reading well" scheme.

5. **Robin Zasio (2011) The Hoarder in You: How to Live a Happier, Healthier, Uncluttered Life.** *New York,* NY: *Random House Press.* This is a self-help book written by a psychologist following his appearance on a US TV programme about hoarding.

6. **Milton Harrison (2020) Hoarding Disorder Help: 15 Minimalist Steps to Help You Declutter.** *Texas: Tower LLC.* This book is written by a New-York-based author who has also released books on drug abuse and anxiety. This was primarily released as an audio book.

7. **Jo Cooke (2021) Understanding Hoarding: Reclaim Your Space and Your Life.** *London: Sheldon Press.* Written by an individual who has worked for various charities and as a civil servant and who supports people affected by hoarding. She is not a clinician. This is a practical book written by someone who has used her personal experience to help others.

8. **Laura Cochran (2021) A–Z of Hoarding: The 7 Reasons People Hoard.** *Create Space Independent Publishing Platform.* This is a book written by someone with experience of hoarding, having grown up in a household with a hoarding parent and having married a hoarder. It is a book which gives advice born from experience.

9. **Pei Nardo (2021) Hoarding Disorder: Recognizing and Understanding Hoarding Disorders: What Hoarding is.** *Self-Published.* This book takes a personal perspective on hoarding and refers to a person who has personal experience of hoarding.

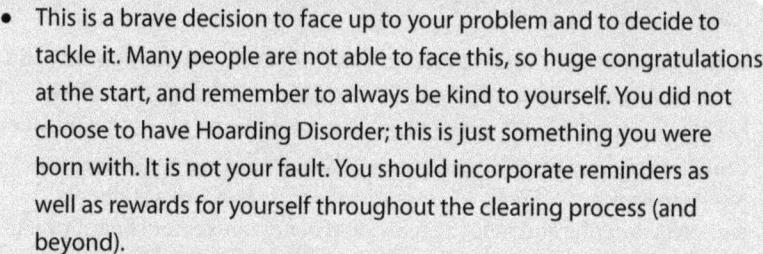

KEY POINTS

- This is a brave decision to face up to your problem and to decide to tackle it. Many people are not able to face this, so huge congratulations at the start, and remember to always be kind to yourself. You did not choose to have Hoarding Disorder; this is just something you were born with. It is not your fault. You should incorporate reminders as well as rewards for yourself throughout the clearing process (and beyond).

- Think about health and safety and any potential risks before starting to clear a hoard, that is, risks of "avalanche", falling, toxic waste, hygiene, pests, etc.

- Some people find it helpful to have a friend/relative helping if possible. This must be a person who is trusted and who will only do what the person with the hoarding problem wishes. It can also be helpful to have support from a local hoarding group. This is not absolutely necessary but can make treatment seem easier.

- A ban on any new items coming into the house throughout the process. This may need some negotiation if an essential item such as food is involved, but none of the types of items previously hoarded should be brought in.

- A maximum of 2 hours a day (can be less) should be dedicated to clearing items. Although it can be tempting to continue, this is emotionally and physically exhausting work, and it is better to apply yourself to short periods where you will not make mistakes and can feel good.

- Choose one room and one area. If there are any safety issues (e.g., blocking of the exit to a property or a fire risk), then this must be tackled first and after a fire risk assessment by the local fire brigade. If no risks, then select an area which will give you the most rewards, for example, clearing the bed to get a good night's sleep, the bathroom so that you can have a long bath once done, etc.

- Stick to this area so that you can really see improvements. It can be tempting to flit from room to room but then it is more difficult to see the progress you are making.

- Once you have decided on an area, then start to divide items into things to keep which have a definite purpose in the near future and those that you will discard. Those discarded items should be put rapidly into black plastic or opaque bags, and once discarded, you should not go back. Once you have sorted the items make sure you take the bags of discarded items to somewhere where you cannot retrieve (i.e., do not leave in the house). It can be useful to have a friend or relative helping at this point who can take them somewhere that you do not know. Similarly, if appropriate, delivering to a charity shop normally means they go to a central depot to be sorted.

- Only handle each article once and make an immediate decision. Even if the decision feels wrong, afterwards it is unlikely to be a "disaster" and you will have a nice tidy home you can enjoy. The longer you hold an item in your hands the more emotionally attached to it you will become. Keep handling to a minimum for this reason.

- Reward yourself as you make progress. Use the money you may have saved from not buying objects to buy a new bath product or to get a special meal, or your reward may be even just to be able to sit in a chair!

- Once you have cleared one area, move on to the next area until the room is cleared. It is then time to repeat the process in another room.

- There will be times when things go wrong. This is to be expected. Be kind to yourself. If it all becomes overwhelming stop for a day or so; remember, this is emotionally and physically draining work, and you need to be really proud of yourself and your achievements. A little slip-up doesn't alter all the good work you have done.

- Good luck. It can seem like a long road ahead but by gradually tackling the problem, you will achieve success.

- It may be helpful for some people to have some professional psychological support that may help you to understand your thinking processes and why you have the problem. This may be available via the NHS or via a number of self-help organisations.

- Finally, remember how brave, courageous, and amazing you are to have faced up to this problem. Well done, and do reward yourself!

11

• • • • • • •

What Can You Do to Help a Friend or Relative Who Has Hoarding Disorder or Hoarding Symptoms?

In this chapter, we examine the difficult problem of trying to offer help and support to a friend or loved one who has Hoarding Disorder. Many people with Hoarding Disorder are reluctant to admit that they have a problem. This may be due to shame and the stigma surrounding the condition or may be due to a lack of insight as the individual has become so accustomed to this way of living and denies there is a problem. Family members and friends need to be empathetic, patient, and tolerant. Constant nagging is likely to increase resistance, so it is a difficult path between urging them to get help but not causing them to feel persecuted and to cut ties with those trying to help them. If their own health and safety, or that of others, is at risk, then we suggest ways in which you can ensure they receive the help they need. At the end of this chapter, we list some of the agencies that can offer help and advice for family, friends, and people living with hoarding problems. While helping a person with hoarding it is imperative you also consider your own health and safety as well as that of the person with hoarding.

Many people with Hoarding Disorder or hoarding symptoms deny that they have a problem. This may be due to the intense shame which they feel in admitting to the problem. If your loved one admits to having a problem, then it is easier for you, but it is still important to recognise how difficult it is for them to admit to the problem due to huge stigma which surrounds this issue. In the past, Hoarding Disorder was not regarded as a mental disorder but was often dismissed as a "lifestyle choice" or was assumed to always be due to another condition, most frequently OCD. Helping someone with Hoarding Disorder requires patience, tact, and compassion towards the individual who is suffering from a difficult and upsetting mental health condition. We have already discussed how people with Hoarding Disorder are frequently depressed and many also suffer from crippling anxiety. Additionally, tragically, almost a quarter of people with Hoarding Disorder attempt to take their own lives. It can be seen how this is a difficult situation and one which should not be dismissed as a minor problem.

First Steps in Helping Someone with Hoarding Disorder

One of the most important things friends and relatives can do for a person with Hoarding Disorder is to offer them a non-judgemental space to talk about their problems. This means understanding about Hoarding Disorder yourself and learning as much as you can about this life-restricting disorder. It is very tempting, but not usually helpful, to rush in and offer immediate advice and urge them to get help for their problems. Many people with Hoarding Disorder have limited insight into their condition, which may have developed over many years, so they are used to living in a crowded and difficult environment. In addition, the stigma surrounding people who do not maintain a clean and tidy home may increase their reluctance to admit to a problem. The subject must therefore be approached gently and with understanding and making clear your wish to help. If you start to criticise or are overly enthusiastic in wanting to sort out the problem, you are more likely to make the person defensive. If you repeatedly mention it, it may be seen as "nagging". So, however difficult, and no matter how desperately you would like to see them living in a neat and clean home, patience is the most important thing to offer. You may raise it and then change the subject to other issues over time. If several family members are concerned, it may be helpful for them to also try to raise the issue. However, this must be done carefully to avoid the person feeling they are being "picked on" by all their family and friends. This may lead to them becoming defensive and refusing to discuss the matter. Some people with Hoarding Disorder have completely cut themselves off from family and friends who have over-enthusiastically tried to intervene.

It is also important to be understanding about the hoarded items. These may look like a pile of rubbish to you but often they are seen as a person's most prized possessions. I was once talking with a lady who had a four-bedroomed house, plus two lockup spaces, rammed ceiling to floor with possessions. Her family had tried to intervene, and she had cut off all contact with them. When I tried to discuss the idea of starting to look at clearing some of these items, she looked at me venomously and stated that what I was suggesting was the same as "raping" her. This shows the extreme attachment people form with their hoarded items.

If it is possible to discuss the hoarding with them, it is worthwhile trying to suggest the advantages of clearing a small area of the living space. For example, pointing out that, if some of the items could be moved from the living room, then family members may visit, etc.

Please take note of the warnings and advice at the end of this chapter regarding you and your loved one's health and safety, and what to think about before visiting their home or intervening in any way.

If there is no way the individual is prepared at this time to consider help for their hoarding behaviour, then more drastic action may need to be considered.

Some of the legal issues have been discussed in Chapter 9. Although it can be extremely difficult to report someone you care about to the authorities, it can be necessary to avoid harm coming to them, their family, neighbours, and members of the public. It is also important, if possible, to maintain a sympathetic ear and offer support to a loved one going through the trauma of some of the interventions which may be necessary. For this reason, it may be better if you can either get others, such as a general practitioner (GP), a religious leader if they have been observant, or a social worker, to do the reporting so that you can step in to offer support.

1. Safety and wellbeing of any children

Children have the right to have a living space which is suitable for them to live, sleep, and play in and not be restricted by excessive clutter. They should also be able to invite friends to their home. If you believe a child's activities are being restricted by a parent's or guardian's hoarding, then there are several steps you can take to help:

- You can contact the local council or a children's charity (in the UK, that is the National Society for the Prevention of Cruelty to Children, NSPCC). This can be done anonymously if necessary.
- Contact the child's GP and report your concerns.
- Contact the child's school to report concerns.
- Document the problem if you can by taking pictures which can be helpful in describing the problem.
- It is important to follow up your actions and to ensure action is being taken by the relevant authorities.

2. Safety of the individual, neighbours, and the public

This topic has been discussed in Chapter 9. What you need to do about this depends on the risk to the individual and their neighbours. It is often easier to get action if a person is living in a flat or apartment than in a detached house.

If the safety of the individual themselves is an issue and they are unwilling to seek help voluntarily, then it may be that you should speak to their GP (with photographs of the problem if possible) and ask them to organise a mental health assessment.

If neighbours or the general public are deemed to be at risk, then contacting the local authority may be the appropriate course of action. They can organise, for example, a fire risk assessment as well as other help.

3. Safety and wellbeing of any pets (animals)

This has been discussed in Chapter 4. Animals should be in a hygienic environment with sufficient room to conduct all their natural behaviours. In the case of any concerns, you can telephone the Royal Society for the Prevention of Cruelty to Animals (RSPCA) anonymously and ask for advice.

Looking after Yourself

If you are helping or visiting a person with hoarding issues, it is extremely important to also take care of yourself and your own health. Make sure you are not placed in any danger from hazards such as:

- Fire with blocked exits
- "Avalanche" of items causing crush injury
- Falls
- Structural damage in the property due to weight of hoarded items
- Damp and mould
- Toxic fumes from stored items
- Risk of infestation and vermin

Visiting someone with severe hoarding requires caution and care and may need old clothes and dust filtering masks to be worn. Overall, if in doubt, do not take risks and call in the experts immediately. Intervening by reporting to the authorities may be detrimental to your relationship, but leaving the individual or placing yourself in danger is potentially much worse than a deterioration in your relationship.

Finally, it can be hugely stressful if you are trying to support and help an individual with Hoarding Disorder, particularly if they are in denial that there is a problem. Make sure you also take care of yourself and your own mental health. If you are struggling and your friend or relative is under the local mental health services in the UK, you can request a carer's assessment for yourself so that any needs you have to be able to continue supporting and caring for your loved one can be addressed. If you do not feel this is necessary, it can still be useful to contact some or one of the charities which deal with hoarding listed below as they can not only offer information and advice but may have support groups specifically aimed at friends, families, and carers.

Useful Telephone Numbers and Websites UK

NSPCC = 0808 800 5000
RSPCA = 0300 1234 999

Organisations that Can Advise on Hoarding Issues in the UK

Hoarding UK

National charity that can provide support, information, and resources for people and families affected by hoarding. As well as advice on treatment and decluttering, they also offer services such as advocacy, etc.

https://hoardinguk.org

OCD Action

National charity that provides help and information for individuals and families affected by Obsessive Compulsive and Related Disorders including Hoarding Disorder.

https://ocdaction.org.uk
0300 636 5478

OCD UK

National charity that provides help and information for individuals and families affected by Obsessive Compulsive and Related Disorders including Hoarding Disorder.

www.ocduk.org
01332 588112 (09:00 – 12:00pm)

Scottish Association for Mental Health (SAMH)

SAMH is the leading mental health charity in Scotland and can offer help and advice for those with Hoarding Disorder and their families. They provide counselling, peer support, and advocacy services.

www.samh.org.uk
0344 800 0550

Northern Ireland Association for Mental Health (NIAMH)

Similar to SAMH, they offer counselling, peer support, and advocacy services.

www.niamhwellbeing.org
028 9032 8474

Local Authorities

Some local authorities have dedicated teams that can offer advice and help to families of hoarders.

Mental Health Services

Mental health services offer treatment and help to individuals with hoarding problems.

Useful Telephone Numbers and Websites in the USA

Child Protective Services (CPS)

A governmental agency.

800-422-4453

National Association of Professional Organizers (NAPO)

An organisation that includes professional organisers that specialise in Hoarding Disorder.

National Center for Hoarding and Cluttering (NCHC)

This is a specialist organisation that offers training, consultancy, and support for professionals and families dealing with Hoarding Disorder. There is information on their website.

Children's Mental Health Services

Contact your local mental health department.

Hoarding Task Forces

Some cities and counties have dedicated task forces.

KEY POINTS

- People with Hoarding Disorder or hoarding symptoms often feel ashamed, humiliated, and embarrassed by their problem.
- Some have little insight and believe their living situation is fine and that others are "picking on them".

- In order to help a family member with hoarding it is important to remain sympathetic, non-judgemental, and patient.
- If the individual wants help, then it can be very helpful for a friend or relative to be involved in the treatment process.
- If they refuse help, then it is essential to consider the health and wellbeing of the individual themselves and others. This includes:
  - Health and wellbeing of any children.
  - Health and safety of the person with the hoarding problem and their safety including risk of fires, falling, etc.
  - Health and safety of neighbours and the public from fires, structural issues, infection, and vermin, etc.
  - Health and wellbeing of any animals kept at the property.
- Whilst helping someone with hoarding problems, it is important to also care for your own health and safety, including your mental health.

Clutter Image Rating

The Clutter Image Rating (CIR) is a tool to help standardise definitions of clutter in the home, created by the International OCD Foundation (IOCDF).[1] It is a pictorial scale ranging from 1 to 9, enabling clinicians, patients, social workers, and other involved parties to look at a room and gauge the level of severity of the hoard objectively. The numbers from 1 to 9 are divided into three sub-groups, 1-3, 4-6, and 7-9. A CIR of 1-3 is considered a "standard living environment", whereas a CIR of 4-6 is cause for concern which will probably require some professional assistance. A CIR of 7-9 is considered severe and requires help and support from multiple agencies for the safety of the patient. However, just because a home may "only" be categorised as a 3 or 4, that does not mean there is not a problem, especially if it's a rapid change from a 1 or 2, for example. If the individual has sought help with hoarding before, it can mean they have identified early on that circumstances have changed or worsened. A home may also vary from room to room, where some may be more or less cluttered than others, so each room must be rated individually.

Below is a short descriptive overview of each level or the Clutter Image Rating, images can be found on the IOCDF website.[2]

Level 1

Level 1 is the lowest level, and this should be a tidy home, with all rooms and furniture able to be used as intended for their purpose. All items should be in an appropriate place, and in good condition. Any collections are categorised.

Level 2

The house is generally tidy; however, some items may be out of place - one or two items of clothing on the floor, newspapers on the sofa, some rubbish left on a table, etc.

Level 3

The house is starting to become messy. There may be more clothing items on the floor, and larger piles of specific items, which are not as easy to keep categorised. An untidy teenager's bedroom would fall under this level!

In this first sub-group of three, all doors and windows are fully accessible, with no blockage. The house will be in good condition, with no obvious issues regarding the maintenance of the property (structural/decorative/the garden, etc.). There will be no unpleasant odour and no pests. Any animals will be well cared for and in suitable numbers.

Level 4

Major furniture will be partially blocked from being used (sofa, bed, bath). All flat surfaces will have clutter. The floor will be visible and usable, but with some trip hazards. The kitchen and toilet will be usable.

Level 5

Inappropriately located items will start "holding up" the hoard, for example, dining table chairs in the bedroom, resulting in blocked pathways. Piles on the floor will now need to be stepped over.

Level 6

Furniture is now almost entirely covered by clutter, except for maybe only the narrowest spaces to sleep or sit. The bathroom is becoming unusable, and it is not safe to cook in the kitchen. The floor is now covered by items.

In this second sub-group of three, at least one major exit to the home will be blocked. The home is starting to become dishevelled and in a state of disrepair. Rooms can no longer be fully used for their purpose. The home may smell of damp, dust, or other slightly unpleasant odours. Any animals may have fleas, be smelly or unkempt, and have toileted indoors. There may start to be infestations of silverfish, excessive spiders, ants, and other insects.

Level 7

The main hoard will be approximately waist height, and the floor is blocked. Narrow pathways have begun to develop between rooms and parts of the hoard. There is no ability to categorise items in a collection.

Level 8

The hoard will be about head height, and dangerous to navigate. Most furniture other than, for example, tall bookcases will not be visible. Windows will mostly be blocked at this point.

Level 9

The hoard is now almost to, or at the ceiling, and is very dangerous to be near.

In this final sub-group, this is severe hoarding. The property will be barely accessible, and the hoard may be visible from outside. There will be significant structural damage from damp, excess weight, and lack of maintenance. Rooms are unusable for almost any purpose. There may no longer be electricity/gas/etc. supplying the property, and the patient will be struggling to maintain personal hygiene. There may be indoor items stored in any outside space, and there may be an unpleasant smell apparent from outside of the property. There will be pest infestations, such as insects, rats, and mice. Any pet animals are in very poor condition and at significant risk.

These highest levels are extremely hazardous, and require multi-agency professional help and guidance, including the mental health team, the fire brigade, environmental health, and other services.

Glossary

Acquisition

This means to obtain by collecting, buying, or being given objects, such as clothes, papers, and other items, or even pets.

Alcohol Misuse Disorders

This refers to the use of alcohol, usually above recommended guidelines which leads to problems in work, home, social leisure, or private leisure activities. It may be that drinking alcohol causes the person difficulty with working, family and friends, ability to self-care, financial difficulties, and even problems with the law.

Recent definition in DSM-5 includes the following possible symptoms and signs:

- Difficulty in controlling or reducing alcohol consumption.
- Drinking more alcohol or for longer than intended.
- Strong desire or craving to drink alcohol.
- Continuing to drink alcohol despite it possibly causing health, relationship, financial, or legal problems.
- Needing increased amounts of alcohol to achieve the desired effect.
- Experiencing withdrawal symptoms such as shaking or nausea and inability to clean teeth due to sickness when alcohol has not been drunk for some time.

Alzheimer's

Alzheimer's is one of the most common forms of dementia and the most common form in old age, although it can also occur in younger persons. This is a progressive disease, and changes usually start slowly but develop over time. Early signs include forgetfulness, difficulty in thinking and working out problems, and sometimes a change in behaviour. Mood changes are also common, with depression being the most common.

Animal Hoarding

This refers to an individual acquiring a larger number of animals than they are able to properly care for. This leads to neglect of the animals. The animals may have been acquired through buying them, being donated them as a form of "rescue", or by the animals breeding. Failure to care adequately for the animals may be due to lack of space, lack of time, and/or lack of money to meet their needs.

Anxiety Disorders

These are a group of disorders where anxiety is the prominent or main symptom. Anxiety occurs in many conditions including depression and OCD, but the term Anxiety Disorders usually refers to one of the following:

- Generalised Anxiety Disorder, whereby an individual experiences almost constant anxiety.
- Panic Disorder, where the individual is consumed by overwhelming panic in certain situations.
- Agoraphobia, which is fear of crowded and enclosed spaces, such as travelling on public transport, visiting busy shops, and stores. This is commonly associated with panic disorder, and in this case is diagnosed predominantly as Panic Disorder.
- Social Anxiety Disorder, which is sometimes referred to as Social Phobia, where the person has problems controlling anxiety when in social situations with other people.
- Specific Phobic Disorder, where people may have fears of specific animals, such as dogs or spiders, or particular situations, such as heights or thunder.
- Separation Anxiety, which is when someone is fearful of leaving friends and family at an age when they would normally be more comfortable with such separations.

Aripiprazole

This is a type of medication which is one of the dopamine blocking drugs. It is commonly referred to as an atypical antipsychotic agent, but the doses used for conditions such as OCD are very much lower than those used in psychotic conditions.

It acts via the brain neurotransmitters of dopamine and serotonin and can, in low doses, be particularly useful in combination with serotonin reuptake inhibiting tablets for OCD and can be helpful in those with Hoarding Disorder.

Arthritis

Arthritis is a general term used to describe pain, inflammation, and stiffness in joints. The most common form is osteoarthritis, which is more common in older age groups. Other types of arthritis include rheumatoid arthritis, which can start in childhood.

Atomoxetine

This medication is particularly useful for children and adults who have ADHD but may have a place in helping those with Hoarding Disorder. It is a selective norepinephrine reuptake inhibitor, which means it works by increasing the levels of the neurotransmitter norepinephrine in the brain.

Attention Deficit Hyperactivity Disorder (ADHD)

This is a condition which starts in childhood (although it can sometimes be diagnosed later in life if overlooked in childhood) and includes symptoms of lack of attention, hyperactivity, and impulsivity. It has been found that many people with ADHD also have significant problems with hoarding.

Autism

The terms Autism and Autistic Spectrum Disorder (ASD) can be used interchangeably. The term ASD is preferable as it emphasises the differences that are found between individuals diagnosed with this condition. This refers to a condition which is present in childhood and features a variety of symptoms having to do with difficulty in social situations, difficulty with communication, and problems with over- or under-sensitivity to sensations, such as sounds, tastes, and textures. The symptoms of autism vary widely from person to person, but key features are:

- Social difficulties. People with autism may struggle with understanding social interactions. This may mean they have difficulty in making and keeping friends, difficulties in understanding other people's emotions and feelings and engaging in two-way conversations.

- Communication issues. Some people with autism have delayed speech and some may never become verbal. Others may have difficulty in understanding "small talk" and may seem brusque or rude as they tell the truth at all times (even when this is upsetting to others).
- Sensory issues. Some people with autism are very sensitive to sensations, such as bright lights or colours, loud sounds, and certain smells, tastes, or textures, which they find unbearable. Others may have a reduced reaction to these senses.

Autistic Spectrum Disorder (ASD)

See above section on Autism.

Body Dysmorphic Disorder (BDD)

This is one of the Obsessive Compulsive and Related Disorders. In BDD, the person is preoccupied with the belief that part of their appearance is ugly or is deformed in some way. They will spend many hours trying to correct this perceived "defect" even though it is not noticeable to others or extremely minor. Hours are spent in front of the mirror and efforts will be made to try to "correct" the perceived defect, for example, wearing heavy make-up, wearing clothes that cover the area, or seeking plastic surgery and even attempting surgery themselves. Most people with BDD also ask for repeated reassurance from people close to them and will usually avoid many social situations or going outside where others can see them without spending many hours on "corrective" procedures. Although it may co-exist with an eating disorder such as Anorexia Nervosa, BDD does not purely focus on weight. It may be linked to perfectionism, as with some other conditions.

Borderline Personality Disorder

See Emotionally Unstable Personality Disorder.

Cerebrovascular Accident (CVA)

This is most commonly referred to as a "stroke". It is the result of a disruption to the blood supply to an area of the brain which causes cells to die in a specific area of the brain. The cause of the disruption to the blood supply is commonly a blockage in one of the blood vessels that feed the brain, but it may sometimes be caused by a bleed which has a similar effect. CVAs can often affect the left hemispheres of the brain and result in speech difficulties as well as right-sided weakness. Even in left-handed people, the speech is often affected in left hemisphere damage.

Citalopram

An antidepressant drug which is known to have specific effects in reducing the symptoms of OCD. It is one of the selective serotonin reuptake inhibiting drugs (SSRIs) and may be helpful for people with Hoarding Disorder.

Clomipramine

The first antidepressant medication to be shown to have specific effects on the symptoms of OCD. Although this is an effective drug in most cases, it also has a large number of side effects. It is a member of the group of medications known as tricyclic antidepressants. Its action in OCD seems to be by increasing the amount of serotonin in the brain. It is known as a serotonin-reuptake inhibitor (SRI) but has largely been succeeded by the selective serotonin reuptake inhibitors (SSRIs), which have fewer side effects in most people. It can be helpful in reducing symptoms in some people with Hoarding Disorder.

Cognitive Behaviour Therapy (CBT)

CBT is a form of therapy whereby the patient's unhelpful and maladaptive thought patterns are identified and then challenged. The challenging is often using behavioural tests or experiments. The amount of the cognitive (working on thoughts) and behavioural (working on actions) components of the therapy can vary greatly. The aim of looking at the thoughts is to change the problematic behaviour. Changing behaviour can often affect the person's thinking about situations without directly challenging the thoughts.

Collection

A collection is a group of objects which bear some similarity to each other, such as a coin collection, a stamp collection, or a record collection. A collection is normally categorised in some way so that, even when there is a huge collection, individual items can be found. For example, a person with a large collection of recipes from newspapers will normally have cut these out of the papers and placed them in folders listing name of the recipe and placed in alphabetical order or by other features which would enable them to be easily found.

Compassion Focussed Therapy (CFT)

This is a therapy which is often described as being a part of the "third wave" or "new wave" of CBT. It was developed by Paul Gilbert and combines elements of CBT with specific interventions aimed to make a person judge themselves with more kindness and compassion. It also uses mindfulness techniques which are based on meditation techniques and focus thinking on the present rather than worrying about the past or the future.

CFT may be useful in people with Hoarding Disorder. It seems to be particularly helpful for people who have problems with shame, have a low opinion of their self-worth, are very self-critical, or who have experienced trauma.

Compulsivity

This refers to the repetitive urge to perform specific actions (or thoughts). These often have ritualistic features and are driven by internal urges or needs. Compulsions frequently have a negative effect on the individual but that does not prevent the urge to perform the compulsive act. As well as the compulsions seen in OCD, compulsions are seen in people with compulsive gambling or compulsive drinking whereby a pattern of behaviour is established in response to certain situations or cues. Compulsivity is different from but can be found in conjunction with impulsivity, which is acting on the spur of the moment in response to situations.

Cost:Benefit Analysis

This entails looking at the costs or down-sides of a particular course of action or behaviour and then considering the benefits of the same. In short, it is weighing up the pros and cons of a situation in a structured way.

D-Cycloserine

This is an antibiotic which was originally developed to treat tuberculosis. It was found, however, to have a beneficial effect on certain learning and memory processes. It has predominantly been used in graded exposure therapy used to treat people with OCD and seems to possibly have a benefit in learning new responses. It may have a role in the treatment of Hoarding Disorder, but there is very little research on this.

Dementia

This is a term which covers a number of conditions and is a general term to describe cognitive decline with reduced memory, thinking, and reasoning for example. Dementia is a progressive disease and is different from brain injury which remains constant. The most common dementia is Alzheimer's dementia.

Depression

This refers to a prolonged low mood which does not improve with an immediate change in circumstances. People have ups and downs in their moods on a regular basis, and these can be in response to bad things happening in their life or their current circumstances. Depression is normally consistent no matter what is happening around the person. A depressed person will not feel happy even if they have received very good news. Some but not all of the most serious depressions are often worse in the early morning and may lift slightly during the day.

Diogenes Syndrome

This is an old-fashioned term which has never been an official diagnosis. It was a term applied to mainly older people who demonstrated extreme hoarding behaviours together with self-neglect and social isolation. It is not a particularly useful term, and nowadays it would be more useful to classify people's difficulties as Hoarding Disorder or one of the other causes of hoarding so that appropriate treatment can be offered.

Dopamine

This is a neurotransmitter or chemical messenger which sends messages from one brain cell to another. Dopamine is associated with feelings of pleasure and also in control of movements. People with the condition of Parkinson's disease have low levels of dopamine in an area of the brain known as the basal ganglia. People with schizophrenia may also have abnormalities in dopamine transmission.

Drug Misuse Disorders

A group of conditions whereby a street drug or a prescribed medication is taken and used to excess. The drug usage often leads to deterioration in the person's ability to work, their relationships with family and others, and their own personal and financial situation. The features of Drug Misuse Disorder are:

- Difficulty in controlling or reducing drug consumption.
- Strong desire or craving to use the drug.
- Continuing to use the drug despite it possibly causing health, relationship, financial, or legal problems.
- Needing increased amounts of the drug to achieve the desired effect.
- Experiencing withdrawal symptoms when the drug has not been used for some time.

Dyscalculia

This is a specific learning difficulty which affects a person's ability to understand numbers and to perform arithmetical and mathematical tasks. It has been described as "number dyslexia". People with dyscalculia are usually of normal intelligence.

Dyslexia

A specific learning disability where, despite normal intelligence, the person has a specific problem with reading, writing, spelling, and sometimes in recognising the sounds in spoken language. It is a very common problem and has been estimated to affect between 5 and 10 per cent of the population. In recent years dyslexia has become much more widely recognised, and specific help can be given to people who have these difficulties to help them to read, write, spell, and punctuate correctly.

Dyspraxia

This is sometimes known as developmental coordination disorder. Dyspraxia may affect a person's ability to make large movements such as difficulties in running, jumping, or riding a bike. It may also affect smaller movements, or there may be problems with hand–eye coordination when a person is seen as "clumsy". It is more widely recognised now than in the past and help can be given. Some people with dyspraxia have problems in planning and performing complex tasks such as following instructions with many stages or in the ability to organise their belongings. It may therefore contribute to hoarding.

Eating Disorders

There are a number of eating disorders, and many may occur in one individual at different times. These range from overeating and obesity, bulimia where large amounts of food are ingested but normal weight is maintained (often by making themselves sick or by prolonged self-starvation after a binge), and anorexia where there is extremely low weight and a low intake of calories. Some people with eating disorders may hoard food either to convince others they are eating it (as in anorexia) or to save up for a "binge". In addition, some people of very low weight do also hoard other items. This association is not well understood but may be a factor of a brain which is being starved of the nutrients it needs to function. The co-existence of anorexia or other eating disorders and Hoarding Disorder is fairly rare but does occur.

Emotionally Unstable Personality Disorder (EUPD)

This is also sometimes known as Borderline Personality Disorder, which is a more old-fashioned term for EUPD. People with EUPD have a history of long-standing inability to regulate emotions. They may experience intense emotions which alter quickly, such as extreme sadness and despair leading to anger and then anxiety and self-dislike. This can lead to self-harming behaviours or an inability to cope with the stresses and strains of life without using alcohol or drugs. The impulsive behaviours can lead to difficulties at work as well as family relationships and even cause them to be in trouble with authorities and the law. Many people with EUPD have a history of trauma in childhood. Many people with EUPD also fear being abandoned and may be excessively clingy or they may push people away from them so that they are the ones in control of abandoning.

Escitalopram

An antidepressant drug which is known to have specific effects in reducing the symptoms of OCD. It is one of the SSRIs and may be helpful for people with Hoarding Disorder.

Fluoxetine

An antidepressant drug which is known to have specific effects in reducing the symptoms of OCD. It is one of the SSRIs and may be helpful for people with Hoarding Disorder.

Fluvoxamine

An antidepressant drug which is known to have specific effects in reducing the symptoms of OCD. It is one of the selective serotonin reuptake inhibiting drugs (SSRIs) and may be helpful for people with Hoarding Disorder. Fluvoxamine was one of the earlier SSRIs to be developed and may have slightly more side effects than the others in some people.

Hair Pulling Disorder

See Trichotillomania.

Hoard

A hoard is an unclassified group of items arranged in an unstructured manner. It is difficult for a person to find a specific item in a hoard. A hoard may consist of one specific type of item or may be a mixture.

Hoarding

Hoarding refers to the excessive accumulation of objects (or sometimes pets) in a way which is out of control and restricts the individual's ability to function in their home (or wherever they keep their hoarded items). People may hoard for a variety of reasons as well as being a feature of Hoarding Disorder.

Hoarding Disorder

Hoarding Disorder refers to the accumulation of a large number of objects which lead to clutter and to which the individual has significant emotional attachment. This behaviour is not better explained by any other medical or mental condition. One of the striking features of Hoarding Disorder is the extreme emotional attachment people with Hoarding Disorder have to their possessions.

Hypomania

This is a mood state where the person has a heightened sense of wellbeing and sometimes irritability. Whereas they may become creative in the early stages of this phase, this rapidly can deteriorate to incompetence. People with hypomania also experience racing thoughts, lack of need to sleep, and general overactivity. Hypomania is a less severe form of mania, where all touch with reality is lost. It is a part of Bipolar Disorder.

Impulse Control

This refers to how we react to our first impulses or how much we act on the "spur of the moment" rather than taking time to think for a while. Obviously not thinking at all before acting can place someone in a dangerous or unwise situation whereas being overly cautious results in someone missing out on opportunities.

Impulsivity

This is the amount of impulse control exhibited by a person. An individual with high impulsivity will take actions leading to immediate sense of reward rather than thinking about what the longer-term effect of these actions may be.

Learning Disability

A person with learning disability may have a specific issue such as dyslexia or "word blindness" or a more universal learning disability. Specific help in areas where learning is difficult can mean that the person reaches their full potential.

Methylphenidate

This is a stimulant which is commonly prescribed to help those with ADHD. Because some people with Hoarding Disorder overlap in their symptoms with ADHD, it may be of help to people with Hoarding Disorder.

Mindfulness

This is a technique derived from the Eastern Buddhist tradition of meditation. In mindfulness, the person is taught to focus on the "here and now" rather than worrying about the past or the future. It involves being in touch with bodily sensations (sight, smell, taste, touch) as well as being aware of emotions and thoughts but observing these rather than being judgemental.

Minocycline

Minocycline is an antibiotic often used to treat bacterial infections but often those of the skin. It has also recently been examined as to whether it has a positive effect in conditions such as Parkinson's disease, rheumatoid arthritis, and multiple sclerosis. As it has actions on the glutamine pathways of the brain, it has been examined as to whether it may have a positive effect in Hoarding Disorder. Very little research, but it is a widely used medication with few side effects and may be helpful to some people with Hoarding Disorder.

Movement Disorder

The term Movement Disorder refers to a group of conditions whereby the person has movements that are either not under their conscious control or are abnormal, has difficulty starting to move, or has problems with controlling their movements. Examples include the tics of Tourette syndrome, the tremor and difficulty starting and stopping in Parkinson's disease, and other neurological and genetic conditions.

Naltrexone

Naltrexone was originally developed for the treatment of opioid addiction (e.g., people who misuse opium, heroin, and over-the-counter medications such as codeine). It acts by blocking the effects of these drugs in the brain and therefore reduces the cravings. More recently, it has been tried in the treatment of people with other impulsive behaviours, such as repeated self-harm, alcohol misuse, and some people with EUPD. It has only been tried in a few people with Hoarding Disorder and is still being researched.

Neurodiversity

This is a concept which defines conditions such as autism, ADHD, dyslexia, dyspraxia, and dyscalculia as being part of the diversity of being human. Rather than referring to these conditions as "disorders", they are seen as on a spectrum of the various human differences in the way our brains work.

Norepinephrine

This is also known as noradrenaline and works both in the brain and also peripherally in the body. In the brain it acts as a neurotransmitter which sends messages between brain cells. It is particularly involved in mood, attention, and degree of arousal. In the body it is secreted by the adrenal glands and is part of the "fight or flight" reaction.

Obsessive Compulsive and Related Disorders (OCaRDs)

This is a new category of conditions included in the *Diagnostic and Statistical Manual of Mental Disorders*, 5th Edition (DSM-5) in 2013. It includes the following

- Obsessive Compulsive Disorder (OCD)
- Body Dysmorphic Disorder (BDD)
- Hoarding Disorder
- Trichotillomania (Hair Pulling Disorder)
- Excoriation Disorder (Skin Picking Disorder)
- OCD related to another medical condition

Obsessive Compulsive Disorder (OCD)

This is a condition that is characterised by horrible, anxiety-producing thoughts, images, or impulses which come constantly into the mind and cause distress. In order to try and control these, the person performs a variety of "putting it right" behaviours or compulsions, such as excessive hand-washing, repeating actions, checking behaviours, as well as repeatedly asking for reassurance. The person also will try to avoid places, situations, or objects which increase these thoughts, so it ends up restricting their functioning at home, at work, and in their social relationships.

Obsessive Compulsive Personality Disorder (OCPD)

This refers to a more persistent state of being meticulous, perfectionistic, and rigid. It may or may not occur together with OCD. Features of OCPD may include:

- Preoccupation with details such as rules, order, organisation, or lists to the extent that the whole point of the activity may be lost and the rules become an end in themselves.
- Perfectionism.
- Overly conscientious and inflexibility in relation to morals, values, and ethics.
- Hoarding of worn-out or worthless objects.
- Reluctance to delegate, as others do not achieve the person's unrelenting standards.
- Miserly approach to spending on self and others.
- Rigidity and stubbornness.

Olanzapine

A type of medication which is one of the dopamine blocking drugs. It is commonly referred to as an atypical antipsychotic agent but the doses used for conditions such as OCD are very much lower than those used in psychotic conditions. It acts via the brain neurotransmitters of dopamine and serotonin and can, in low doses, be particularly useful in combination with serotonin reuptake inhibiting tablets for OCD and can be helpful in those with Hoarding Disorder.

Paralysis

A condition characterised by a loss of function in the muscles of part of the body. There are many possible causes including a stroke, by brain or spinal cord injury, by a progressive neurological condition such as motor neurone disease, or some people are born with paralysis. The muscles involved vary according to the cause and where the damage to the brain, spinal cord, or peripheral nerves is located.

Paroxetine

An antidepressant drug which is known to have specific effects in reducing the symptoms of OCD. It is one of the SSRIs and may be helpful for people with Hoarding Disorder.

Perpetuating Factors

Situations, events, or other factors which maintain a behaviour once it has developed.

Personality Disorders

A group of mental health conditions which normally arise during adolescence or early adult life. These conditions are characterised by enduring patterns of thoughts, behaviours, and/or feelings which result in difficulties in achieving the person's life aims, and usually cause difficulty in functioning in a number of areas and cause the individual distress.

Personality Disorders are more long-standing than most acute mental health problems and appear to be part of the individual's personality. However, these conditions can be helped, usually with psychological therapies, if the person wants to change problematic patterns of behaviour.

Post-Traumatic Stress Disorder (PTSD)

A condition which arises following trauma, such as being involved in or witnessing an accident, a crime, war, or other traumatic events. These traumatic events may involve the individual themselves or they may witness others being harmed or maimed. Features of PTSD are:

- **Intrusive thoughts** which include recurrent and distressing thoughts and memories concerning the traumatic event. These include "flashbacks" where the person feels temporarily transported to the place of the trauma and "witnesses" it again in their mind's eye. In addition, people often have recurring nightmares, repetitive thoughts, and extreme distress concerning the trauma.
- **Hyperarousal** whereby the person is permanently "on edge" and overly vigilant looking for another traumatic event to happen. The person may have anger outbursts, difficulty sleeping, and an exaggerated startle response to minor incidents.
- **Avoidance** of people and places which remind them of the original trauma.
- **Changes in thinking and mood** where the person generally has low mood and may view themselves and others in a negative way.

Precipitating Factors

The factors which directly cause the symptoms to first emerge. For example, it may be that an individual has a strong family history of depression and may be prone to develop this, but it may be the death of a loved one or the loss of a job which causes the depression to arise.

Predisposing Factors

These are the factors which make a person more likely to have a particular condition. This does not mean that developing the condition is inevitable but that it is more likely. Examples include genetic factors with a family history of a particular condition or the circumstances of early life, such as living in poverty, etc.

Psychoeducation

This means explaining and teaching a person about mental health conditions and how their condition may have arisen within their particular circumstances. It aims to inform the person about their condition and, thereby, help them to move forward in their own treatment and recovery.

Psychosis

This refers to a group of conditions where a person loses and becomes out of contact with a sense of reality. Symptoms may include hearing voices when there is no one there, having the experience that the television or radio is directly referring to them, having abnormal beliefs or "delusions" about situations. Abnormal beliefs have to be compared with the person's religion and cultural beliefs before being labelled as delusions. For example, I may not believe that little green men are walking around the countryside, but within some sectors of society, this may be considered a normal belief.

Psychotic

This refers to psychosis. Someone may be described as psychotic if they lose contact with reality in deeply held conviction.

Quetiapine

A type of medication which is one of the dopamine blocking drugs. It is commonly referred to as an atypical antipsychotic agent, but the doses used for conditions such as OCD are very much lower than those used in psychotic conditions. It acts via the brain neurotransmitters of dopamine and serotonin and can, in low doses, be particularly useful in combination with serotonin reuptake inhibiting tablets for OCD and can be helpful in those with Hoarding Disorder.

Relapse Prevention

This refers to planning to help a person recognise the individual signs of relapse in themselves and to make plans as to what are the best courses of action to take at these early stages to prevent a full-blown recurrence of the problem.

Risperidone

A type of medication which is one of the dopamine blocking drugs. It is commonly referred to as an atypical antipsychotic agent, but the doses used for conditions such as OCD are very much lower than those used in psychotic conditions. It acts via the brain neurotransmitters of dopamine and serotonin and can, in low doses, be particularly useful in combination with serotonin reuptake inhibiting tablets for OCD and can be helpful in those with Hoarding Disorder.

Selective Serotonin Reuptake Inhibitors (SSRIs)

These are a group of medications which act by increasing serotonin in specific areas of the brain. They are citalopram, escitalopram, fluoxetine, fluvoxamine, paroxetine, and sertraline. They are known as SSRIs as their action is focussed on serotonin rather than other neurotransmitters.

Senile Dementia

This is a progressive disease which starts in older age in which changes usually start slowly but develop over time. Early signs include forgetfulness, difficulty in thinking and working out problems, and sometimes a change in behaviour. Mood changes are also common, with depression being the most common. It is often referred to as Alzheimer's as the areas of the brain affected are identical to those seen in this condition.

Serotonin

This is a neurotransmitter which transmits messages and signals between nerve cells. It seems to be the major neurotransmitter involved in depression, OCD, and anxiety.

Serotonin Norepinephrine Reuptake Inhibitors (SNRIs)

As the name suggests, these medicines work by increasing the levels of the neurotransmitters (chemical messengers) serotonin and norepinephrine in the brain. SRIs remain the medication of choice for OCD and SNRIs are not indicated for these people. However, there is growing evidence which seems to support SNRIs in the treatment of Hoarding Disorder.

Serotonin Reuptake Inhibitors (SRIs)

These are a group of medications which include the SSRIs and also clomipramine. As an older type of drug known as a tricyclic antidepressant, clomipramine works predominantly via serotonin but is not as specific as the SSRIs.

Sertraline

An antidepressant drug which is known to have specific effects in reducing the symptoms of OCD. It is one of the SSRIs and may be helpful for people with Hoarding Disorder.

Skin Picking Disorder

Skin Picking Disorder is sometimes called Excoriation Disorder or dermatillomania and is one of the Obsessive Compulsive and Related Disorders. It involves picking of the skin, and the urge to do so tends to build until the picking is performed which provides short-lived relief from the build-up of tension. In addition, many people also skin pick when distracted and not paying attention. It can cause problems with infection and may need medical treatment for this.

Stigma

This is the negative attitudes, beliefs, and stereotypes which individuals or society may hold against people with certain characteristics. Mental disorders of all types are often stigmatised, but this has been very marked with relation to people with Hoarding Disorder, who have been portrayed as being dirty and lazy rather than the truth that they are people who have a mental health condition and require help to deal with this. Stigma often prevents people coming forward for help as they fear the reaction of other people.

Trichotillomania

This is also known as Hair Pulling Disorder. It is one of the Obsessive Compulsive and Related Disorders. It involves pulling out of the hair, often in one particular spot, but it can be all over the head, face, and body. People describe a growing urge to pull out hair which is only very temporarily relieved by doing so. Some people also hair pull when not fully aware they are doing this. Large bald areas or general lack of hair can be the result as well as specific hair loss due to plucking eyelashes, pubic hair, etc.

Venlafaxine

This is one of the serotonin norepinephrine reuptake inhibiting medications. It is mainly used in depression, generalised anxiety, social anxiety, and panic disorders but has been suggested as a useful medication for some people with Hoarding Disorder.

Resources

Information Sources

National Health Service (NHS) has information about hoarding. Available at: www.nhs.uk/mental-health/conditions/hoarding-disorder

Royal College of Psychiatrists has online information for people with hoarding and their families and friends. Available at: www.rcpsych.ac.uk/mental-health/mental-illnesses-and-mental-health-problems/hoarding#:~:text=If%20it%20is%20a%20symptom,better%20with%20just%20psychological%20therapy

British Psychological Society has a leaflet on hoarding. Available at: https://cms.bps.org.uk/sites/default/files/2024-05/Understanding%20Hoarding%20-%20Information%20Leaflet.pdf

British Journal of General Practice has recently published guidelines for general practitioners (family doctors) on helping people with hoarding problems. Available at: https://bjgp.org/content/73/729/182

Self-Help Organisations

There are some organisations which deal exclusively with hoarding, and many of the self-help organisations dealing with Obsessive Compulsive and Related Disorders also have considerable experience in hoarding and have offered help, support, and advice to many individuals affected by hoarding over the years.

Hoarding UK: Support for people affected by hoarding, including support groups. Available at: info@hoardinguk.org; https://hoardinguk.org/

OCD Action: UK-based organisation providing support as well as information and meetings for people living with OCD and related disorders, including hoarding; their relatives, friends, and carers. Available at: www.ocdaction.org.uk

OCD-UK: UK-based organisation providing support as well as information and meetings for people living with OCD and related disorders, including hoarding; their relatives, friends, and carers. Available at: www.ocduk.org

Orchard OCD: UK-based charity that also has links with the USA and other international groups working with OCD and related disorders, including hoarding. This charity works to accelerate the development of new and better treatments for these conditions. Available at: www.orchardocd.org

TOP UK: UK-based organisation offering support and treatment groups for people with phobic anxiety, OCD, and related disorders. Available at: www .topuk.org

International OCD Foundation: US-based organisation offering conferences and information for people with OCD and related disorders (including hoarding) and also professionals. Available at: https://iocdf.org

SANE: Australian-based charity for mental health offering information and forums for conditions including OCD and related disorders. Available at: www.sane.org/information-and-resources/facts-and-guides/ obsessive-compulsive-disorder

Other Organisations

International College for Obsessive Compulsive Spectrum Disorders (ICOCS): An international organisation which sets out to promote research in OCD and related disorders and to produce public statements to improve OCD treatment internationally. Available at: www.icocs.org

International OCD Foundation: US-based organisation aiming to promote awareness about OCD and related disorders, promote research, and provide information to professionals and people with OCD and related disorders. Available at: https://iocdf.org

Role of Decluttering Services

Many independent companies have been set up in recent years as there is increased awareness of the problem of hoarding. Some of these have been sub-contracted by the NHS as well as housing associations and local councils. Whereas a decluttering service may be necessary in an acutely dangerous situation to ensure the safety of the person with hoarding problems and their family and neighbours, it will generally only provide a temporary solution. Unless the underlying hoarding behaviours are addressed, then it is inevitable that the problem will recur in a few months or years.

For this reason, we would advise that any decluttering services are used in combination with treatment of the underlying condition.

Further Reading

1. **Gail Steketee and Christina Bratiotis (2020)** *Hoarding: What Everyone Needs to Know.* **New York: Oxford University Press.**

   This is a book written by clinicians and experts in the field of hoarding who explain how to recognise hoarding problems and discuss psychological and community treatment.

2. **David F. Tolin, Randy O. Frost, and Gail Steketee (2014)** *Buried in Treasures: Help for Compulsive Acquiring, Saving, and Hoarding.* **Second Edition. New York: Oxford University Press.**

   This is a self-help book written by clinicians and experts in the field. It is a practical guide and is particularly useful for people who wish to start tackling hoarding problems.

3. **Satwant Singh, Margaret Hooper, and Colin Jones (2015)** *Overcoming Hoarding: A Self-Help Guide Using Cognitive Behavioural Techniques.* **London: Robinson.**

   This book is part of the "Overcoming" series, which publishes self-help books in the UK for predominantly a UK market. Many of these titles have been placed on the "Reading well" scheme.

4. **Jo Cooke (2021)** *Understanding Hoarding: Reclaim Your Space and Your Life.* **London: Sheldon Press.**

   Written by an individual who has worked for various charities and as a civil servant, and who supports people affected by hoarding.

5. **Laura Cochran (2021)** *A–Z of Hoarding: The 7 Reasons People Hoard.* **Create Space Independent Publishing Platform.**

   This is a book written by someone with experience of hoarding, having grown up in a household with a hoarding parent and having married a hoarder. It is a book which gives advice born from experience.

6. **Pei Nardo (2021)** *Hoarding Disorder; Recognizing and Understanding Hoarding Disorders: What Hoarding Is.* **Self-published.**

This book takes a personal perspective on hoarding and refers to a person who has personal experience of hoarding.

7. **Bowe Packer (2014)** *Compulsive Hoarding: Understanding and Treating Compulsive Hoarding.* **Create Space Independent Publishing Platform.**

This book is written by a man who has published over 25 self-help books on a variety of subjects in the USA.

Notes

1. Introduction

1. Shackle, S. 4 July 2023. "You reach a point where you can't live your life." What is behind extreme hoarding? *Guardian Newspaper.*

2. BBC News. 21 December 2017.

3. Akinci, M.A., Turan, B., Esin, I.S., et al. Prevalence and correlates of hoarding behavior and hoarding disorder in children and adolescents. *European Child and Adolescent Psychiatry.* 2022;31:1623–34.

2. When Does Hoarding Arise?

1. Neary, D., Snowden, J.S., Gustafson, L., et al. Frontotemporal lobar degeneration: a consensus on clinical diagnostic criteria. *Neurology.* 1998;51(6):1546–54. doi: 10.1212/wnl.51.6.1546

2. Lebert, F. Diogenes syndrome, a clinical presentation of fronto-temporal dementia or not? *International Journal of Geriatric Psychiatry.* 2005;20(12):1203–4. doi: 10.1002/gps.143020,1203120416315145

3. Hoarding Disorder

1. Shackle, S. 4 July 2023. "You reach a point where you can't live your life" What is behind extreme hoarding? *Guardian Newspaper.*

2. BBC News. 21 December 2017.

4. Animal Hoarding

1. David, J., Crone, C., Norberg, M. A critical review of cognitive behavioural therapy for hoarding disorder: how can we improve outcomes? *Clinical Psychology and Psychotherapy.* 2022;29:469–88.

2. Animal welfare crisis warning over cost of living. BBC News. 25 July 2023. www.bbc.com/news/uk-scotland-66300806

5. Obsessive Compulsive Disorder, Obsessive Compulsive Personality Disorder, Hoarding Disorder, and How They Interact

1. *Diagnostic and Statistical Manual of Mental Disorders*, 5th ed., Text Revision (DSM-5-TR). Washington, D.C.: American Psychiatric Association. 2022.
2. Pinto, A, Teller, J. and Wheaton, M.G. Obsessive compulsive personality disorder: a review of symptomatology, impact on functioning, and treatment. *Focus*. 2022;20(4):389–96.

8. Treatment of Hoarding Disorder: Psychological Approaches

1. Frost, R.O., Steketee, G. *Stuff: Compulsive Hoarding and the Meaning of Things*. New York, NY: Houghton-Mifflin Harcourt. 2010.
2. Chou, C., Tsoh, J.Y., Shumway, M., et al. Treating hoarding disorder with compassion-focused therapy: a pilot study examining treatment feasibility, acceptability, and exploring treatment effects. *British Journal of Clinical Psychology*, 2020;59(1):1–21. https://doi.org/10.1111/bjc.12228

Clutter Image Rating

1. https://hoarding.iocdf.org/professionals/clinical-assessment/
2. https://hoarding.iocdf.org/wp-content/uploads/sites/7/2016/12/Clutter-Image-Rating-3-18-16.pdf

Index